# Communication Sciences
# Student Survival Guide

This guide is dedicated to students in communication sciences and disorders programs who are trying to figure out what to do to survive.

—*Marie Patton*

This guide is dedicated to my family, especially my parents and sister, who have been so supportive throughout my journey of becoming an SLP. To my friends at Augie and WSU who I have continuously recruited to volunteer for various projects concerning NSSLHA. Also, to all of those amazing professors and supervisors who have guided me through my education of becoming an SLP, and specially Karen Mahan, who encouraged me to join national NSSLHA my freshmen year of college.

—*Carol Hassebroek*

# Communication Sciences
# Student Survival Guide

## SECOND EDITION

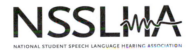

NATIONAL STUDENT SPEECH LANGUAGE HEARING ASSOCIATION

Edited by Carol A. Hassebroek, B.A.

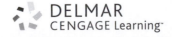

DELMAR
CENGAGE Learning™

Australia • Brazil • Japan • Korea • Mexico • Singapore • Spain • United Kingdom • United States

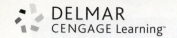

## DELMAR
### CENGAGE Learning

Communication Sciences Student Survival Guide, 2nd edition

NSSLHA

Edited by Carol A. Hassebroek

Vice President, Career and Professional Editorial: Dave Garza

Director of Learning Solutions: Matthew Kane

Senior Acquisitions Editor: Sherry Dickinson

Managing Editor: Marah Bellegarde

Product Manager: Laura J. Wood

Editorial Assistant: Anthony Souza

Vice President, Career and Professional Marketing: Jennifer Ann Baker

Marketing Director: Wendy E. Mapstone

Senior Marketing Manager: Kristin McNary

Marketing Coordinator: Scott A. Chrysler

Production Director: Carolyn Miller

Senior Art Director: David Arsenault

For product information and technology assistance, contact us at **Cengage Learning Customer & Sales Support, 1-800-354-9706**

For permission to use material from this text or product, submit all requests online at **www.cengage.com/permissions.** Further permissions questions can be emailed to **permissionrequest@cengage.com**

Library of Congress Control Number: 2009933912

ISBN-13: 978-1-4354-8102-2

ISBN-10: 1-4354-8102-X

**Delmar**
5 Maxwell Drive
Clifton Park, NY 12065-2919
USA

Cengage Learning is a leading provider of customized learning solutions with office locations around the globe, including Singapore, the United Kingdom, Australia, Mexico, Brazil, and Japan. Locate your local office at: **international.cengage.com/region**

Cengage Learning products are represented in Canada by Nelson Education, Ltd.

To learn more about Delmar, visit **www.cengage.com/delmar** Purchase any of our products at your local college store or at our preferred online store **www.ichapters.com**

**Notice to the Reader**

Publisher does not warrant or guarantee any of the products described herein or perform any independent analysis in connection with any of the product information contained herein. Publisher does not assume, and expressly disclaims, any obligation to obtain and include information other than that provided to it by the manufacturer. The reader is expressly warned to consider and adopt all safety precautions that might be indicated by the activities described herein and to avoid all potential hazards. By following the instructions contained herein, the reader willingly assumes all risks in connection with such instructions. The publisher makes no representations or warranties of any kind, including but not limited to, the warranties of fitness for particular purpose or merchantability, nor are any such representations implied with respect to the material set forth herein, and the publisher takes no responsibility with respect to such material. The publisher shall not be liable for any special, consequential, or exemplary damages resulting, in whole or part, from the readers' use of, or reliance upon, this material.

Printed in the United States of America
1 2 3 4 5 6 7 13 12 11 10 09

# Contents

# Preface

*Communication Sciences Student Survival Guide* is a must-have resource for individuals considering a career in communication sciences and disorders (CSD) as audiologists, speech–language pathologists, or speech–language–hearing scientists. By providing practical advice from CSD students and professionals, this text enables users to learn everything from differences in CSD degrees, to how to choose and get into the right educational program, to how to be successful as an undergraduate, graduate student, and professional. In addition, mentors of students in CSD will find this text to be a valuable resource for its many tips and tricks, including student checklists, listing of related professional associations, with pertinent Web sites, and suggested readings.

## REASON FOR THIS GUIDE

This project started as a booklet that the National Student Speech Language Hearing Association's (NSSLHA) executive council sought to create to meet the needs of NSSLHA members. When Marie A. Patton, the first editor, was a regional councilor during her junior year of college, she read a proposed table of contents and began brainstorming other topics that would be useful and thought provoking. Months later, she read the draft of the document, which included approximately 10 pages of advice for undergraduates and master's students. The draft was a great start, but it needed more advice and content areas. So more material was added, and through invitation, students from various universities reviewed the document and offered suggestions. Moreover, an active dialogue was initiated; ultimately, other content areas such as advice for doctoral students, why is it important to take both audiology and speech–language pathology (SLP) courses, clinical fellowships, and the job outlook were added. The NSSLHA executive council and director of operations Dawn Dickerson also provided invaluable feedback and contributed to the growing document. Approximately 3 years after Marie Patton's initial effort, with the assistance of over 150 students and professionals, the guide became a reality.

During the spring 2008 NSSLHA executive council meeting, the executive council decided to revise the guide. Carol Hassebroek, a current regional councilor, along with Dawn Dickerson, director of operations, began revising the guide. Many chapters were combined and revised, and with the assistance of many CSD students and professionals, new chapters were added.

# HOW THIS TEXT IS ORGANIZED

*Communication Sciences Student Survival Guide* is divided into five sections: (1) Information About the Professions, (2) Year-by-Year Guides, (3) Advice for Special Populations, (4) The Basics of Money, Research, Writing, and Interviews, and (5) Professional Associations.

The first section, Information About the Professions, addresses such basic questions as:

- Who is an audiologist?
- What does a speech–language pathologist do?
- What does the job market look like for individuals with different CSD degrees?
- What is the importance of shared audiology and speech–language pathology courses?

The next section, Year-by-Year Guides, provides advice specific to individuals at different points in their CSD education—from high school through Ph.D.

The section Advice for Special Populations provides advice for:

- Parents
- Adults returning to college to pursue a CSD degree
- Students from culturally and linguistically diverse backgrounds
- Students with an undergraduate degree in another discipline
- U.S. and international students studying abroad

The fourth section, The Basics of Money, Research, Writing, and Interviews, contains:

- Advice on financing your CSD education
- Research basics
- Advice on writing a thesis
- Advice on writing for the clinical practicum
- Advice for seeking a job, through résumé and interview preparation

The final section, Professional Associations:

- Explains how NSSLHA is organized and operates
- Explains how to attend American Speech–Language–Hearing Association conventions
- Contains interviews with Special Interest Division coordinators about how they became interested in their content area
- Contains a listing of professional organizations that are of interest to CSD students and professionals

The appendices offer a variety of useful tools.

- Appendix A lists materials that can assist individuals in being organized.
- Appendix B provides a list of suggested reading related to CSD.
- Appendix C lists key acronyms and phrases that students encounter in the field (e.g., *ASHA, IEP, CF,* and *Au.D.*); however, this appendix does not include acronyms of diagnoses and treatments because they are beyond the scope of this guide.

In addition to the appendices, throughout the book there are helpful checklists and top ten from the NSSLHA Now! newsletters.

## HOW TO USE THIS GUIDE

The unique advantage of this book is that it does not have to be read from front to back. It is designed for individuals to access information as needed throughout their academic journey. For example, an individual who is just considering a career in CSD might begin with Chapters 1 and 2. These chapters explain the professions of audiology and speech–language pathology and how promising the job outlooks are. Depending upon an individual's place in life (e.g., college student, postbachelor's, nurse, engineer), the reader can look in the table of contents for the advice chapter that best applies.

Once an individual reads the chapter, or chapters, that most directly applies to him or her, subsequent advice chapters can be read to prepare for the next academic step (e.g., sophomores can read the junior, senior, and master's/doctoral chapters). Reading these chapters will assist a student in knowing what to expect in his or her academic future.

A useful feature of this guide are the worksheets, checklists, and top-10s included in some chapters. You may photocopy these tools for personal use; they are intended to help organize important information.

Mentors, including faculty members, NSSLHA leaders, high school guidance counselors, and any individual who might want to be a mentor, would benefit from reading this guide. Mentors and guidance counselors can share the ideas that would be helpful to students considering and/or studying CSD and design their mentoring or guidance programs to reflect this advice.

Of course, reading the entire book will help one get the most complete picture of the academic requirements and the profession as a whole, but this guide can be tailored to meet any individual's needs.

## AVENUE FOR FEEDBACK

Anyone who has questions, suggestions, or comments about the guide can contact the NSSLHA National Office at nsslha@asha.org. NSSLHA welcomes students who have more advice and experiences to share for the guide. NSSLHA and the editor hope *Communication Sciences Student Survival Guide* provides you with support, advice, and encouragement, and wish you the best of luck in your academic programs and your professional career.

## ABOUT THE EDITOR, CAROL A. HASSEBROEK, BA

Carol Hassebroek is currently working on her master's of arts in speech–language pathology at Wichita State University in Wichita, Kansas. She completed her bachelor's of arts in communication sciences and disorders at Augustana College in Sioux Falls, South Dakota, in 2004. Carol has been actively involved in NSSLHA since her freshman year at Augustana College when she joined both her local chapter and the national association. Her energetic participation in NSSLHA has led to greater involvement with professional CSD organizations on the local, state, and national levels.

Carol's interest in the discipline began during her senior year of high school after her mother, a school secretary, had talked to the school speech–language pathologist about the profession and encouraged Carol to study the CSD discipline in college. She declared CSD her major before starting college. Carol knew she wanted to be a speech–language pathologist after taking the introduction to CSD course at Augustana. In her junior year of college, she served her local NSSLHA chapter as treasurer and was elected on the NSSLHA executive council as the region 6 representative. During Carol's senior year, she continued to serve NSSLHA as her local chapter's vice president and on the executive council. Since being elected to the executive council, she has severed on ASHA's Board of Division Coordinators and on ASHA's 2009 convention program committee under the interest topic of Language and Infants, Toddlers, and Preschoolers. Carol has spoken to students about NSSLHA at two state conventions, and she has attended four ASHA conventions. In 2009 Carol was elected to serve a second term on the NSSLHA executive council.

As a graduate student, Carol continues to be active in her local NSSLHA chapter and works as a graduate research assistant under Dr. Antje Mefferd, Ph.D, CCC-SLP. Carol plans to eventually return to school for a Ph.D.

## ABOUT THE PREVIOUS EDITOR, MARIE A. PATTON, BHS

Currently, Marie Patton is a master's student in speech–language pathology at the University of Wisconsin–Madison. She completed her bachelor's of health sciences in communication disorders at the University of Kentucky, in Lexington, Kentucky. She not only has experience as a student in CSD but has experience with student and professional organizations at the local, state, and national levels.

Marie knew she wanted to be a speech–language pathologist during high school when she read about the profession at a local public library and then observed a speech–language pathologist (Francine Emmons). As a freshman in college, she joined the University of Kentucky's NSSLHA chapter and continued her membership until graduation. During her sophomore year, Marie was elected regional councilor for the NSSLHA executive council. Moreover, she volunteered at the Kentucky Speech–Language–Hearing Association's office in Lexington, Kentucky. During her junior year, Marie was elected the president of NSSLHA. As part of this position, she was a voting member on the ASHA legislative council. During the spring of her junior year, she started working on this guide and continued to add to the text each semester, as she gained more advice from peers and had more experiences. During her senior year, Marie was the editor of the local NSSLHA chapter's newsletter.

As a graduate student at the University of Wisconsin–Madison, Marie has been a member of the local NSSLHA chapter and the editor of the newsletter. She has spoken at four state conventions and two teleseminars on topics related to leadership and advice for students. Most recently, Marie has attended five state conventions and three ASHA conventions. She is also a project assistant and has an interest in augmentative and alternative communication. After graduation, Marie plans to work for a few years before returning to school for a Ph.D.

# Contributors to the First Edition

Marie A. Patton, BHS
  *Communication Sciences Student Survival
  Guide* Editor and Coordinator
  NSSLHA President, 2002–2003; NSSLHA
  Regional Councilor, 2001–2003; ASHA
  Legislative Councilor, 2002–2003
  Graduate student in speech-language
  pathology at the University of Wisconsin-
  Madison

Nichole Castle
  Graduate student in speech-language
  pathology at Eastern Washington
  University

Michelle Cox, MA, CCC-SLP
  Doctorate of Philosophy candidate in
  Composition Studies at the University
  of New Hampshire

Lee Cruz
  Assistant Director of Placement Services in
  Counseling and Career Services at Saint
  Xavier University

Vicki Deal-Williams, MA, CCC-SLP
  ASHA Chief Staff Officer for Multicultural
  Affairs

Dawn D. Dickerson, MPA
  NSSLHA Director of Operations

Erica Dmuchoski, BS
  NSSLHA Regional Councilor, 2001–2003;
  ASHA Council on Clinical Certification,
  2002
  Au.D. candidate at Central Michigan
  University

Kelly Farquharson
  NSSLHA Regional Councilor, 2003–2005
  Graduate student in speech-language
  pathology at Pennsylvania State University

Larissa Fedak, BS
  NSSLHA Regional Councilor, 2002–2004
  Graduate student in special education at New
  Jersey City University

Jeremy Federman, BS
  NSSLHA Regional Councilor, Region III,
  2003–2005
  Graduate student in hearing sciences at
  Vanderbilt University

Cynthia Gannett, Ph.D.
  Director of Writing Across the Curriculum at
  Loyola College

Jeanette Glenn, BS
  Graduate student in audiology at the
  University of Wisconsin-Madison

Sharon Goodson, MS, CCC-A
  NSSLHA President, 2000–2002; NSSLHA
  Regional Councilor, Region X, 2000–2002;
  ASHA Legislative Councilor, 2001–2002
  Graduated from San Francisco State University

Caryn Neuvrith, BS
  NSSLHA President, 2003–2004; ASHA
  Legislative Councilor, 2003–2004
  Sc.D. candidate in audiology at Seton
  Hall University

Kristi L. Pennypacker, BS
  Graduate student in speech-language
  pathology at Bloomsburg University

Amy Solomon Plante, MEd, CCC-SLP
Clinical Assistant Professor at the University
of New Hampshire

Jeremy Saylor
Undergraduate in speech-language pathology
at the University of Kentucky

Jeanne O'Sullivan, MEd, CCC-SLP
Clinical Assistant Professor at the University
of New Hampshire

Sheri Tracy
Graduate student in speech-language
pathology at the University of Wisconsin-
Madison

Sherri Webster, BA
Graduate student in speech-language
pathology at Western Washington
University

# Contributors to the Second Edition

Carol Hassebroek, BA
Communication Sciences Student Survival
Guide, 2 nd ed. Editor
NSSLHA Regional Councilor, Region VI,
2007–2011; ASHA Board of Division
Coordinators, 2008–2009
Graduate student in speech-language
pathology at Wichita State University

Ahmad Alexander
Contributor: Advice for the Audiology
Externship
Reviewed: Importance of Shared Audiology &
Speech-Language Pathology Courses

Virginia Best
Author: CSD Professional Associations

Marilyn Burns, Certification Case Manager, ASHA
Author/Contributor: Figure 11–2 Tips for
completing the application for certification

Kimberly Croteau, AuD, CCC-A
Contributor: Advice for the Audiology
Externship

Kristi Degenhardt
Reviewed: Advice for Students with an
Undergraduate Degree in Another
Discipline

Vickie B Dionne Au.D. CCC-A
Contributor: Advice for the Audiology
Externship

Laura Dosher
Reviewed: Introduction to the Professions

Marilyn Dunham Wark, MA, CCC-SLP
The University of Memphis
Reviewed: Resumé and Interview Preparation
and Advice for Parents

Melissa R Eldred
Reviewed: Advice for Students from Culturally
and Linguistically Diverse Backgrounds

Lanee Friedel, MS, CCC-SLP/A
Authored: Advice for Parents

Kate Foenander BA/BSc, DipAud, MAudSA
Doctor of Audiology Student
AAA; NAFDA; ASHA; NSSLHA member
Member of the Audiological Society of
Australia
Golden Key International Honour Society
Contributor: Advice for the Audiology
Externship

Angelica Gunn
Reviewed: Advice for First-Year Graduate
Students

MaryKate Harwood
Reviewed: Advice for Freshman Year,
Sophomore Year, Junior Year, Senior Year

Kylie Hockenberry
Reviewed:
Introduction to the Professions
Doctoral Degrees and Applying to a Doctoral
Program
Being Active in the American Speech-
Language-Hearing Association

Dan Hudock
Reviewed: Job Outlook and Salary
Expectations

Silvia Martinez, EdD, CCC-SLP
Reviewed: Doctoral Degrees and Applying to
Doctoral Programs

Christine Neumayer
Reviewed: Adults returning to college

Amanda Norris
Contributor: Professional Associations
in Communication Sciences

Sue Postelwait
Reviewed:
Advice for First-Year Graduate Students
Advice for Second-Year Graduate Students
Doctoral Degrees and Applying to a Doctoral
Program
Information about Post-Doctorates
Author: Advice for Choosing a Clinical
Fellowship in Audiology and Speech-
language Pathology

Katie Quinlan, AuD, CCC-A
Contributor: Advice for the Audiology
Externship

Roger Reeter
Reviewed:
Financing your CSD Education
Advice for High School Students
Advice for Undergraduate Students
Advice for Adults Returning to College to
Pursue a CSD Degree
Advice for Students from Culturally and
Linguistically Diverse Backgrounds
Advice for Students with an Undergraduate
Degree in Another Discipline

Sara Robinson
Reviewed:
Advice for Senior Year
Transitioning from Undergraduate to Graduate
Coursework
Research Basics
Writing a Thesis
Writing for the Clinical Practicum

Leigh Anne Roden
Author: Advice for the Clinical Practicum
Reviewed: Writing for the Clinical Practicum

Lyndsey Seeley
Reviewed: Transitioning from Undergraduate
to Graduate Coursework and Advice for
1st year Graduate students

Sally Smith
Reviewed: Financial Aid

Tejwatie Sohan
Contributed: Extracurricular/Leadership
Activities NSSLHA/ASHA Allows Students

Susan Yao-Tresguerres
Reviewed:
Other Career Options in CSD
Doctoral Degrees and Applying to a Doctoral
Program

Aynsley Warden
Contributor: Advice for US and International
Student Studying Abroad

Rosaline Zelkin
Reviewed: Selected Specialty Interests
in Speech-Language Pathology

# Acknowledgments

Thank you to all students and professionals who contributed to this book. A special thank you to Dawn Dickerson, NSSLHA Director of Operations, for all of her diligent work and input that she added to this book.

*—Carol Hassebroek*

I would like to thank every student and professional who has assisted with this book. I would especially like to thank Dawn Dickerson, NSSLHA Director of Operations, and Larissa Fedak, NSSLHA Regional Councilor, who spent many long days and nights assisting me in completing various drafts of this guide. I would like to thank Mary Fleming, who assisted me in writing the proposal to Delmar Learning for this book.

*—Marie Patton*

## REVIEWERS

On behalf of Delmar Cengage Learning, we would like to thank the following content reviewers for their valuable feedback during the development process:

Erin Davlin
4th year AuD student
Ohio University
Athens, OH

Daniel J Hudock M.S., Doctoral Student
1st year Doctoral Student, Research Assistant
East Carolina University
Greenville, NC

Gina Nalesnik
NSSLHA Vice President
Regional Councilor, Region 1
Master's Student in Speech Language Pathology
The Pennsylvania State University
University Park, PA

Gayle B. Neldon, MS, CCC/A
Hearing Clinic Coordinator
West Virginia University Dept. of Speech
    Pathology & Audiology
Morgantown, WV

Colleen M. O'Rourke, Ph.D.
Associate Professor and Program Coordinator
Georgia State University
Atlanta, GA

# PART 1

## Information about the Professions

# CHAPTER 1

# Professions in Communication Sciences and Disorders

## INTRODUCTION

A career in audiology and speech–language pathology is incredibly rewarding and exciting. By assessing, treating, and researching speech, language, and hearing disorders, audiologists and speech–language pathologists (SLPs) positively impact the lives of individuals with communication challenges and their families. The American Speech–Language–Hearing Association (ASHA) certifies these professionals as clinicians once they complete academic coursework, clock a specified number of supervised clinical practicum hours, and pass The Praxis Series examination in audiology or speech–language pathology administered by the Educational Testing Service (ETS).

This chapter briefly examines the professions that make up communication sciences and disorders. Moreover, this chapter is an excellent starting point for anyone interested in learning more about the professions.

## WHAT IS COMMUNICATION SCIENCES AND DISORDERS?

The discipline of communication sciences and disorders encompasses a wide variety of problems in speech, language, and hearing. Professionals in this discipline are audiologists, SLPs, and speech and hearing scientists. These professionals diagnose, treat, and research a variety of hearing, speech, and swallowing disorders in newborns, children, adults, and the elderly. (Source: http://www.worldwidelearn.com/online-education-guide/health-medical/communication-disorders-major.htm)

Communication disorders come in different forms and affect all races, ages, and ethnicities. Some disorders are genetic, and others may develop as a result of a physical trauma (e.g., paralysis) or as part of the natural aging process (e.g., hearing loss in the elderly).

With such a wide range of people afflicted by communication disorders, professionals in this field enjoy a tremendous opportunity to specialize. Some SLPs and audiologists focus on diagnosing or treating infants born with communication disorders, and others concentrate on preventing the degradation of elderly patients' abilities to communicate. Below is more information about the professions of audiology and speech–language pathology, where they practice, and the specific disorders that they are certified to treat.

# WHAT IS AUDIOLOGY?

Audiology is the study of the diagnosis, treatment, and prevention of hearing and balance impairments. Audiologists are professionals trained to treat people of all ages with hearing loss.

Audiology is an attractive career because it is so diverse. In addition to treating hearing loss, audiologists are responsible for dispensing hearing aids and developing treatments to prevent hearing loss. Audiology is an ideal career for those who want to improve the quality of life of individuals with hearing and balance impairments. Audiologists can also teach at universities to help students gain knowledge and obtain their degrees and certifications. Moreover, they can be hearing scientists who conduct research in hearing and design hearing equipment. Many audiologists are involved in a combination of these pursuits and may engage in research, clinical work, and instruction all at once. Within the field, an audiologist can specialize in the following areas, among others:

- **Auditory processing disorders.** Specialists in auditory processing disorders focus on acoustical signal processing in the peripheral and central auditory systems.
- **Auditory–verbal therapy.** Auditory–verbal therapy focuses on, among others, early identification of hearing loss and the promotion of auditory discrimination and language comprehension (i.e., following cochlear implant surgery). Moreover, an auditory–verbal therapist is an audiologist or an SLP who imparts the skills necessary to use this therapy at home to caregivers (usually family members) of a person with a hearing impairment.
- **Cochlear implants.** Cochlear implants are hearing devices surgically implanted into ears to improve hearing. The audiologist, in conjunction with a team of other medical professionals (i.e., SLPs; ears, nose, and throat doctors; psychologists), is responsible for diagnosing the degree and type of hearing loss and assessing speech perception skills and tonal thresholds, and is actively involved throughout the rehabilitation of patients with hearing disorders.
- **Audiology professors.** Audiologists in this area work for an institute of high education conducting research and providing instructions to future audiologists and SLPs.
- **Geriatric audiology.** Geriatric audiology involves diagnosing hearing disorders and providing appropriate rehabilitation for the elderly with hearing impairments.
- **Intraoperative monitoring.** Intraoperative monitoring involves monitoring a patient's hearing by using electrophysiological testing during an operation.
- **Occupational audiology.** Occupational audiology involves preserving hearing in settings where there is possible harmful noise exposure, and studying the treatment and prevention of hearing loss and hearing conservation in industrial settings.

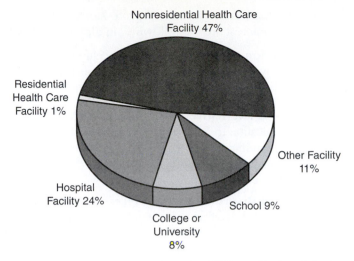

**Figure 1-1** Primary employment settings for ASHA-certified audiologists *(Source: ASHA Summary Membership and Affiliation Counts, 2007 year-end)*

- **Pediatric audiology.** Pediatric audiology involves screening, diagnosing, and treating hearing loss in children. A pediatric audiologist also provides information on educational placements for children focusing on sign language and deaf culture.
- **Vestibular disorders.** Specialists in vestibular disorders treat auditory nerve disorders affecting balance.

In addition to the many areas of specialization, audiologists work in a variety of settings. Figure 1-1 graphically represents the primary employment settings for ASHA-certified audiologists. These settings include the following:

- Corporations and nonprofit organizations
- Colleges and universities
- Hospitals
- Private practices
- Rehabilitation clinics
- Schools

## WHAT IS SPEECH–LANGUAGE PATHOLOGY?

Speech–language pathology is the study of the diagnosis, treatment, and prevention of disorders that affect speech, language, and swallowing. Speech, language, and swallowing are activities that are vital to daily living, and when impaired, these activities have a large impact on an individual's quality of life.

Similar to audiology, speech–language pathology is appealing as a career because it is diverse. An SLP can work with people of all ages, with a variety of special populations, and in a multitude of professional settings. Some of the most common areas of interest are the following, in alphabetical order:

- **Accent modification.** Often, to help them modify their accent through articulation therapy, individuals learning English as a second language choose to seek the services of an SLP.

- **Augmentative and alternative communication (AAC).** AAC provides a means of communication to individuals who are unable to independently and efficiently communicate verbally because of a limitation. Examples of AAC are sign language and a portable computerized device with speech output.

- **Autism spectrum disorders (ASD).** ASD is a spectrum of developmental disabilities that affect verbal and nonverbal communication and social interaction. SLPs assist individuals with ASD with their social communication skills.

- **Child language.** Child language specialists are involved in examining children's ability to properly formulate speech/language and express themselves verbally. SLPs work with children who may say only a few or no words to improve their intelligibility, word choice, vocabulary, sentence structure, and social communication skills.

- **Cleft palate and craniofacial disorders.** Cleft palate and craniofacial disorders are congenital conditions involving craniofacial structural anomalies. For example, cleft palate is a hole in the hard or soft palate (the roof of the mouth). Cleft palate causes a distortion of speech because it allows extra airflow from the mouth or nose. As a result, the speech of individuals with cleft palate may sound breathy or nasal.

- **Disfluency (also known as *stuttering*).** Disfluency refers to the inability of speech to flow. Currently, the cause of stuttering is not known; however, SLPs are an important part of ongoing research in this area.

- **Dysphagia.** Dysphagia, difficulty in swallowing, is a swallowing disorder that may be caused by weakness in the muscles used for swallowing, paralysis of the vocal folds, stroke, or other neurogenic disorders.

- **Neurogenic speech and language disorders.** Neurogenic speech and language disorders occur because of injury to the brain (before, during, or after birth). One common example of neurogenic speech and language disorders often seen by SLPs is aphasia, the inability to understand and/or express language.

- **Voice disorders.** Specialists in voice disorders work with impairments at the level of the larynx (i.e., vocal folds) caused by misuse, neurogenic conditions, or external trauma. SLPs working in voice disorders may also work with professional voice users such as singers and actors.

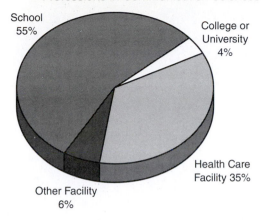

**Figure 1-2** Primary employment settings for ASHA-certified speech–language pathologists *(Source: ASHA Summary Membership and Affiliation Counts, 2007 year-end)*

These areas of interest are by no means an exhaustive list in speech–language pathology. Figure 1-2 provides the primary employment settings for ASHA-certified speech–language pathologists. There are multiple settings in which an SLP can work:

- Acute care and rehabilitation hospitals
- Public and private schools
- Colleges and universities
- Corporations and nonprofit organizations
- Private practices
- Research labs
- Skilled nursing facilities and assisted living facilities

## CONCLUSION

As can be seen from the abundance of options for an audiologist or an SLP, these careers can lead to a diverse and rewarding professional life. The discipline is constantly changing, and new research is always being conducted. Today's research leads to new assessment and treatment options for individuals with communication disorders tomorrow. Within communication sciences and disorders, anyone who wants to make a difference in the lives of others can find a niche in audiology or speech–language pathology.

# CHAPTER 2

# Job Outlook and Salary Expectations

## INTRODUCTION

One of the pressing concerns among students choosing a major is whether it will land them a job after graduation. For many students, it is important not only to do something enjoyable but also to find a job that pays well. Certainly, given the expense of obtaining an undergraduate or a graduate degree, you should know whether, ultimately, you will be able to achieve your personal goals and financially support yourself. This chapter discusses the job outlook for audiologists and speech–language pathologists (SLPs) and presents mean salaries for each profession. The good news is that, for audiologists and SLP, the job market looks very promising! As with most professions, an individual's earning potential depends on many factors, including personal motivation; area of specialization; where in the country you work; whether you work for a private practice, a not-for-profit clinic, or a research university; and how much you work (full time, part time, or in an educational setting with summers off). Though there are many variables, the mean salaries discussed in this chapter provide a good idea of the expected salary ranges.

## EMPLOYMENT OUTLOOK FOR AUDIOLOGY AND SPEECH–LANGUAGE PATHOLOGY

According to the *Occupational Outlook Handbook* of the U.S. Department of Labor, Bureau of Labor Statistics, the job outlook for audiology and speech–language pathology is promising. Essentially, the elderly population is rapidly increasing. This increase is, in part, due to the baby-boom generation reaching middle age and medical advances that have increased the survival rate of trauma and stroke victims. With the increasing elderly population and medical advances, employment opportunities in health and rehabilitation services are on the rise. For example, hearing loss is strongly associated with aging, so an aging population will create more jobs for audiologists. Likewise, as the older population increases, the incidence of cerebrovascular accidents (strokes) will likely rise, and the need for SLPs in rehabilitation clinics and hospitals will increase.

The need for the communication sciences and disorders (CSD) professional is not limited to the aging populations. Employment for CSD professionals is on the rise as public and health care professionals have become more aware of the importance of identifying and diagnosing hearing, speech, and language problems early. Moreover, anticipated growth in elementary, secondary, and special education enrollments will create more job opportunities in schools. The fact that federal law guarantees special education and related services to all qualified children (i.e., children with speech, language, and/or hearing disorders [*Occupational Outlook Handbook*]) will ensure that there is an increase in job opportunities for CSD professionals who work with these children.

In addition, schools, hospitals, and nursing facilities are increasingly using contract services to hire CSD professionals, as well as there is an increased demand for direct services to clients. These developments will increase the number of audiologists and SLPs choosing to work in, or run, private practices. There is also a shortage of qualified personnel in inner cities and the rural and less populated areas of the United States (*Fact Sheet: Speech-Language Pathology*). All this means more opportunities for individuals with CSD degrees.

Figures 2-1 through 2-3 offer a more detailed look at salaries by profession, employment facility, academic degree, years of experience, and geographic region.

(a)

| Employment Facility | Median Calendar Year Salary | | | |
|---|---|---|---|---|
| | 1995 | 2000 | 2004 | 2006 |
| School | $40,244 | $48,000 | $65,000 | $68,000 |
| College/university | $41,000 | $52,000 | $63,000 | $69,000 |
| Hospital | $43,000 | $48,000 | $64,000 | $65,000 |
| Residential health care facility | $42,000 | $n = <25$ | $n = <25$ | $n = <25$ |
| Nonresidential health care facility | $38,117 | $45,000 | $60,000 | $63,000 |
| Private physician's office | $36,000 | $43,000 | $55,500 | $60,000 |
| Other nonresidential health care facility | $38,000 | $48,000 | $62,000 | $69,250 |

*Note:* $n = 714$ (1995); $n = 719$ (2000); $n = 915$ (2004); $n = 1,160$ (2006).
*Source:* 1995 and 2000 ASHA Omnibus Surveys and 2004 and 2006 ASHA Audiology Surveys.

*(continues)*

**Figure 2-1** Median calendar year salaries of audiologists by (a) primary employment facility, (b) level of academic degree, (c) years of experience, and (d) geographic region

(b)

| Academic Degree | Median Calendar Year Salary | | | |
|---|---|---|---|---|
| | 1995 | 2000 | 2004 | 2006 |
| Master's | $40,000 | $46,000 | $58,116 | $60,000 |
| Doctorate | $63,000 | $70,000 | * | * |
| Au.D. | * | * | $65,000 | $68,000 |
| Ph.D. | * | * | $82,606 | $90,000 |

*Item not included in survey.
*Note:* n = 800 (1995); n = 862 (2000); n = 912 (2004); n = 1,148 (2006).
*Source:* 1995 and 2000 ASHA Omnibus Surveys and 2004 and 2006 ASHA Audiology Surveys.

(c)

| Years of Experience | Median Calendar Year Salary | | | |
|---|---|---|---|---|
| | 1995 | 2000 | 2004 | 2006 |
| 1–3 | $30,000 | $36,000 | $45,000 | $52,000 |
| 4–6 | $34,000 | $42,000 | $50,000 | $54,000 |
| 7–9 | $40,000 | $45,000 | $59,780 | $60,000 |
| 10–12 | $40,000 | $48,000 | $61,155 | $63,879 |
| 13–15 | $43,000 | $52,500 | $60,000 | $65,000 |
| 16–18 | $50,000 | $60,000 | $62,095 | $68,000 |
| 19–21 | $52,000 | $57,500 | $70,002 | $69,595 |
| 22–24 | $50,000 | $60,000 | $72,564 | $79,000 |
| 25–27 | $60,000 | $60,000 | $72,734 | $78,809 |
| ≥28 | $51,000 | $64,500 | $78,000 | $80,000 |

*Note:* n = 804 (1995); n = 648 (2000); n = 913 (2004); n = 1,155 (2006).
*Source:* 1995 and 2000 ASHA Omnibus Surveys and 2004 and 2006 ASHA Audiology Surveys.

(d)

| Geographic Region | Median Calendar Year Salary | | | |
|---|---|---|---|---|
| | 1995 | 2000 | 2004 | 2006 |
| Northeast | $43,000 | $48,000 | $65,000 | $70,000 |
| Midwest | $39,050 | $45,000 | $57,000 | $60,000 |
| South | $40,000 | $46,750 | $60,000 | $63,000 |
| West | $42,000 | $54,000 | $66,890 | $68,000 |

*Note:* n = 801 (1995); n = 865 (2000); n = 911 (2004); n = 1,157 (2006).
*Source:* 1995 and 2000 ASHA Omnibus Surveys and 2004 and 2006 ASHA Audiology Surveys.

**Figure 2-1**  (*Continued*)

(a)

| Practice Setting | Median Calendar Year Salary | |
|---|---|---|
| | 2005 | 2007 |
| Overall | $60,000 | $65,000 |
| General medical hospital | $61,250 | $65,000 |
| Rehabilitation hospital | $58,920 | $60,500 |
| Pediatric hospital | $60,000 | $60,000 |
| Skilled nursing facility | $68,200 | $75,000 |
| Home health agency or client's home | $53,000 | $57,500 |
| Outpatient clinic or office | $60,000 | $63,000 |

*Note:* n = 630 (2005); n = 648 (2007).
*Source:* 2005 and 2007 ASHA SLP Health Care Surveys.

(b)

| Years of Experience | Median Calendar Year Salary | |
|---|---|---|
| | 2005 | 2007 |
| 1–3 | $52,694 | $51,500 |
| 4–6 | $51,850 | $56,450 |
| 7–9 | $53,730 | $62,086 |
| 10–12 | $58,000 | $65,000 |
| 13–15 | $62,000 | $65,000 |
| 16–18 | $67,000 | $64,000 |
| 19–21 | $65,000 | $80,000 |
| 22–24 | $70,000 | $69,840 |
| 25–27 | $70,000 | $74,400 |
| ≥ 28 | $78,146 | $74,000 |

*Note:* n = 619 (2005); n = 648 (2007).
*Source:* 2005 and 2007 ASHA SLP Health Care Surveys.

(c)

| Geographic Region | Median Calendar Year Salary | |
|---|---|---|
| | 2005 | 2007 |
| Northeast | $60,000 | $65,532 |
| Midwest | $60,000 | $62,000 |
| South | $58,000 | $65,000 |
| West | $68,000 | $70,000 |

*Note:* n = 628 (2005); n = 648 (2007).
*Source:* 2005 and 2007 ASHA SLP Health Care Surveys.

**Figure 2-2** Median annual salaries of health care–based speech–language pathologists by (a) practice setting, (b) years of experience, and (c) geographic region

(a)

| School Setting | Median Academic Year Salary | | |
|---|---|---|---|
| | **2004** | **2006** | **2008** |
| Overall | $50,000 | $52,131 | $58,000 |
| Day or residential | $46,000 | $60,128 | $64,932 |
| Preschool | $48,500 | $53,290 | $57,008 |
| Elementary | $50,000 | $52,000 | $57,000 |
| Middle, junior high, or secondary | $53,000 | $54,750 | $60,840 |
| Combined (several) | $48,500 | $51,537 | $58,000 |
| Other | $56,000 | $62,500 | * |

*Item not included in survey.
*Note:* "Overall" includes respondents who did not indicate a school setting. $n = 1,987$ (2004); $n = 1,669$ (2006); $n = 1,636$ (2008).
*Source:* 2004, 2006, and 2008 ASHA Schools Surveys.

(b)

| Years of Experience | Median Academic Year Salary | | |
|---|---|---|---|
| | **2004** | **2006** | **2008** |
| 1–3 | $38,669 | $40,041 | $n < 25$ |
| 4–6 | $39,500 | $43,000 | $46,254 |
| 7–9 | $42,500 | $44,000 | $49,000 |
| 10–12 | $45,000 | $46,000 | $52,000 |
| 13–15 | $48,250 | $50,000 | $55,000 |
| 16–18 | $52,250 | $53,000 | $57,138 |
| 19–21 | $50,100 | $58,000 | $61,060 |
| 22–24 | $55,800 | $60,000 | $63,000 |
| 25–27 | $57,000 | $60,000 | $62,977 |
| ≥ 28 | $60,000 | $64,900 | $65,000 |

*Note:* $n = 1,985$ (2004); $n = 1,668$ (2006); $n = 1,633$ (2008).
*Source:* 2004, 2006, and 2008 ASHA Schools Surveys.

*(continues)*

**Figure 2-3** Median academic year salaries of school-based speech–language pathologists by (a) primary school setting, (b) years of experience, and (c) geographic region

(c)

| Geographic Region | Median Academic Year Salary | | |
|---|---|---|---|
| | 2004 | 2006 | 2008 |
| New England | $54,000 | $60,000 | $61,000 |
| Mid-Atlantic | $61,000 | $65,000 | $68,900 |
| East North Central | $51,000 | $55,000 | $60,000 |
| West North Central | $44,000 | $47,000 | $49,000 |
| South Atlantic | $47,000 | $48,000 | $55,000 |
| East South Central | $41,000 | $43,180 | $49,500 |
| West South Central | $41,494 | $43,000 | $48,000 |
| Mountain | $48,000 | $50,000 | $55,000 |
| Pacific | $60,000 | $64,802 | $63,000 |

*Note: n* = 1,978 (2004); *n* = 1,660 (2006); *n* = 1,634 (2008).
*Source:* 2004, 2006, and 2008 ASHA Schools Surveys.
Geographic regions with corresponding states

| New England | CT, ME, MA, NH, RI, VT |
|---|---|
| Mid-Atlantic | NJ, NY, PA |
| East North Central | IL, IN, MI, OH, WI |
| West North Central | IA, KS, MN, MO, NE, ND, SD |
| South Atlantic | DE, DC, FL, GA, MD, NC, SC, VA, WV |
| East South Central | AL, KY, MS, TN |
| West South Central | AR, LA, OK, TX |
| Mountain | AZ, CO, ID, MT, NV, NM, UT, WY |
| Pacific | AK, CA, HI, OR, WA |

**Figure 2-3** (*Continued*)

## CONCLUSION

Discussions of this chapter can be boiled down to a few important facts: Students interested in helping individuals with communication and hearing challenges can look forward to not only making a positive impact on the lives of their clients but also finding rich opportunities in a healthy job market. In addition, they can expect to make a comfortable living.

## REFERENCES

American Speech-Language-Hearing Association. (n.d.). *Fact sheet: Audiology.* Retrieved July 9, 2009, from http://www.asha.org/careers/professions/overview/audiology.htm.

American Speech-Language-Hearing Association. (n.d.). *Fact sheet: Speech-language pathology.* Retrieved July 9, 2009, from http://www.asha.org/careers/professions/overview/slp.htm.

Ghazzawi, G. (2008, August 20). Annual, hourly salary figures available: Salary results of the 2003 ASHA Omnibus Survey released. *The ASHA Leader,* pp. 1–10.

U.S. Department of Labor, Bureau of Labor Statistics. *Occupational outlook handbook, 2008–09 edition: Audiologists.* Retrieved July 9, 2009, from http://www.bls.gov/oco/ocos085.htm.

U.S. Department of Labor, Bureau of Labor Statistics. *Occupational outlook handbook, 2008–09 edition: Speech-language pathologists.* Retrieved July 9, 2009, from http://www.bls.gov/oco/ocos099.htm.

# CHAPTER 3

# The Importance of Shared Audiology and Speech–Language Pathology Courses

## INTRODUCTION

For their undergraduate coursework in communication sciences and disorders, audiology students take some speech–language pathology-oriented courses and, likewise, speech–language pathology students take some audiology-oriented courses. Therefore, they may wonder why they share the same major with students who have different career goals. The American Speech–Language–Hearing Association (ASHA) is home to the credentialing agency that certifies professionals in audiology and speech–language pathology. One of the requirements for certification is that students majoring in audiology complete classes and clock a specified number of clinical hours in speech/language rehabilitation. Similarly, speech–language pathology majors must complete classes and clock a specified number of clinical hours in hearing/aural rehabilitation. Although audiology and speech–language pathology are two separate professions within CSD, both audiologists and speech–language pathologists (SLPs) assess, diagnose, and treat individuals with communication disorders. Understanding why and how the professions work together is an important function of working effectively as an audiologist or an SLP.

## WHY SHARE COURSEWORK?

The following are some of the reasons why future audiologists and speech–language pathologists (SLPs) share the same coursework:

- Hearing, speech, and language are intricately related. Both audiologists and SLPs need a comprehensive understanding of human development, anatomy, and the communication process.

- An audiologist may work with children with receptive language disorders. An audiologist who has a background in speech and language rehabilitation will be able to understand the client's needs and adjust their language so that they, in turn, will understand the tasks necessary for a hearing evaluation. Also, SLPs may work with clients who have hearing loss and/or auditory processing disorders. SLPs who work with older adults with voice, swallowing, speech, and/or language disorders are likely to have clients with hearing loss due to aging. As a result, to assess their hearing, SLPs may refer their clients to audiologists.

- SLPs need to rule out hearing loss as a possible cause or factor in a client's speech or language disorder. An SLP may have difficulty providing treatment to a child or adult with an untreated hearing loss. The client is likely to struggle in understanding the SLP without a hearing aid, sign language, or other adaptive strategies that may be recommended by an audiologist. An SLP should be competent in basic hearing screening.

- On multidisciplinary teams, audiologists and SLPs work together in evaluating patients. Knowing more about the other's scope of practice is an added advantage for diagnosing and treating patients with communication disorders.

- CSD professionals work together with individuals who may require cochlear implants. Audiologists complete evaluations for the implant, and SLPs teach speech to these clients after the implantation.

- Because SLPs are likely to work with clients with hearing aids, they should know how hearing aids work and how to replace a battery and adjust the volume in some hearing aid models.

As you continue your study, you will discover more ways the professions are interrelated.

## WORKING TOGETHER TO IMPROVE EFFECTIVENESS

The following list provides some suggestions on how future audiologists and SLPs can work together to improve the effectiveness of treatment given to clients.

- If you are an audiologist seeing a child client with a hearing impairment, screen the client's speech and language. If speech and/or language pathology exists, refer your client to an SLP. Similarly, if you are an SLP seeing a child client with speech–language pathology, screen the client's hearing. If an untreated hearing impairment exists, refer your client to an audiologist.

- If you are an audiologist treating an adult who has had a stroke, has suffered traumatic brain injury (TBI), or has other neurological deficiencies, consider referring the adult to an SLP, based on what you know about the characteristics of speech and language disorders. If you are a speech–language pathologist who has an adult client with TBI, aphasia, or other neurological deficits, consider referring the client to an audiologist, based on what you know about the characteristics of hearing loss.

- If you are an audiologist, know at least one SLP who works with children and adult clients, so you can contact the SLP when you have pertinent questions about a client with a speech and/or language disorder. If you are an SLP, know at least one audiologist who works in diagnostics and aural rehabilitation, so you can contact the audiologist when a client has a possible hearing loss or when you are uncertain about a type of aural rehabilitation treatment.

- Lobby Congress about bills that will affect the CSD discipline as a whole. ASHA members have access to the advocacy Web page that lists current legislative issues Congress is considering related to these professions. In the Web page, the members can also find the contact information for congresspersons. Visit the legislation and advocacy page of the ASHA Web site regularly and stay informed about issues impacting the professions. Advocacy is key to ensuring that our careers and clients are protected.

## CONCLUSION

Audiologists and speech–language pathologists share more than coursework and the common goal of helping individuals with communication disorders. ASHA accredits colleges and universities through the Council of Academic Accreditation on Audiology and Speech-Language Pathology. This large professional organization provides certification, continuing education, support, and services to individuals working in the CSD discipline, thus furthering the close association between audiologists and SLPs that begins with shared undergraduate coursework and continues through professional practice.

# PART 2

## Year-by-Year Guides

# CHAPTER 4

# Advice for High School Students

## INTRODUCTION

If you are a high school student interested in a career in audiology or speech–language pathology, you will find this chapter guiding you through what you can do before you start college. Read on for tips on how to figure out whether communication sciences and disorders (CSD) is the career path for you, how to prepare for college, and how to find a college that offers a major in audiology and speech–language pathology. Moreover, Figure 4-1 provides a handy checklist of things to do to help you prepare for this next step.

☐ Learn more about what audiologists and speech–language pathologists do.

☐ Job shadow a local audiologist, speech–language pathologists, or speech–language–hearing scientist.

☐ Keep track of hours you spend observing an audiologist or speech–language pathologist.

☐ Keep your science notes.

☐ Take courses in science that will prepare you for college.

☐ Take writing courses.

☐ Make sure the colleges/universities you apply to have a CSD program.

☐ Visit a National Student Speech Language Hearing Association (NSSLHA) chapter.

☐ Visit the CSD department where you are applying to college.

☐ Order a complimentary subscription to NSSLHA's newsletter.

☐ Get involved.

☐ Consider working part-time.

☐ Volunteer.

**Figure 4-1** Checklist for high school students interested in a CSD undergraduate degree *(Source: Delmar/Cengage Learning.)*

## LEARN MORE ABOUT WHAT AUDIOLOGISTS AND SPEECH–LANGUAGE PATHOLOGISTS DO

To make informed decisions about where you want to go to school and what you want to spend your time studying, you must learn as much as you can about the professions. Most libraries have books on health care professions, such as *Introduction to the Health Professions, Fifth Edition* (Peggy S. Stanfield, Nanna Cross, and Y. H. Hui, Jones and Bartlett Publishers, 2009). You may also find books on sign language, Deaf culture, disabilities, hearing loss, stuttering, autism, hearing aids, and other topics related to communication disorders. Spending some time at your local library can really help you understand what a career in CSD could mean for you. There are also many excellent novels and guidebooks related to CSD that you may like to read. (See Appendix B for suggestions.)

Another great place to learn more about the professions is the Internet. For example, the Student sections of the National Student Speech Language Hearing Association (NSSLHA) and American Speech–Language–Hearing Association (ASHA) Web sites have current information about issues in the professions.

## JOB SHADOW A LOCAL AUDIOLOGIST, SPEECH–LANGUAGE PATHOLOGIST, OR SPEECH–LANGUAGE–HEARING SCIENTIST

Job shadowing provides you an opportunity to follow a professional during a typical day at work. By job shadowing, you get to see firsthand what the typical day of a professional is like and you can decide whether a career in audiology or speech–language pathology is really right for you.

Audiologists and speech–language pathologists (SLPs) work in various settings, including hospitals; speech and hearing clinics; and elementary, middle, and high schools. To locate an audiologist or an SLP, look in the phone book for a clinical practice, call a local hospital and ask to speak with the audiologist or SLP, or contact your guidance office and ask if your school district has an audiologist or an SLP on staff or on call. You may also ask your family members and friends if they know any professional audiologist or SLP. Sometimes, a personal reference can help you get your foot in the door.

When you speak with the audiologist or SLP over the telephone, you may want to say the following: "I am a student at ——— High School. I am interested in becoming an audiologist/speech–language pathologist. If you have time, I would like to come in to briefly talk with you about the profession and to possibly observe your day at work."

When you meet with the audiologist or SLP, you should dress professionally. Wear a nice pair of pants and a dress shirt or sweater; wearing jeans and a T-shirt would be inappropriate. Ask the audiologist or SLP what the dress code is for their particular place of employment (i.e., in a hospital you may be asked to wear scrubs). Depending on the setting, there may be a specific dress code that you will need to observe. Be respectful of the professional you are meeting with and the patients or clients you may come into contact with. If someone has kindly agreed to take time out of his or her busy workday to meet with you, the impression you make can influence his or her decision to meet with other high school students interested in job shadowing.

To make the most of your time with the audiologist or SLP, you should prepare questions ahead of time and bring a pen and a notebook to take notes. Some questions you may want to ask are:

- What do you do here? What's a typical day like?
- What do you like best about your job?
- What do you find to be the most challenging part of your job?
- Have you worked in different settings? What do you like about the settings you have worked in? What have you not liked?
- What advice do you have for students interested in this profession?
- Where did you receive your degree, and how did your education process go?

Moreover, you may also ask which topical journals to review during downtime while shadowing. Looking at current literature can help you visualize what it means to keep up to date while you are still practicing in the field.

After you meet with or observe the audiologist or SLP, ensure that you send a thank-you note. Although a thank-you e-mail is thoughtful, an actual thank-you note received via mail makes a much better impression. If you are interested in continuing your research into the field, mention that you would be interested in volunteering. Ask if the audiologist or SLP knows of any opportunities; you want to establish good relationships early. If you have the opportunity to work as a volunteer with a professional, you may want to call on him or her in the future for a reference or a letter of recommendation.

## KEEP TRACK OF HOURS YOU SPEND OBSERVING AN AUDIOLOGIST OR A SPEECH–LANGUAGE PATHOLOGIST

Some undergraduate programs may be interested in learning how many observational hours you have logged with an audiologist or an SLP. Your time observing while in high school can give you a jump on your preparation for the professions. Most important, the hours observed in high school are separate from those required for ASHA certification. The observation hours required by ASHA will probably be addressed in your undergraduate program during your junior and/or senior years. For your personal information, keep a folder, binder, or computer record of all the time you spend observing an audiologist or an SLP. You should also keep contact information of all individuals you observed or volunteered with. Make sure that you have their name, address, telephone number, and e-mail address, and the name of their practice, company, hospital, or employer.

## KEEP YOUR SCIENCE NOTES

College-level communication sciences classes reintroduce many of the research practices that you learn in high school biology and anatomy classes. Therefore, you keep your science notes from high school. You will need this information in the future. For example, some colleges may require a physics of sound class. If you keep notes from previous physics or science classes, you can spend less time reviewing and more time learning new information.

## TAKE COURSES IN SCIENCE THAT WILL PREPARE YOU FOR COLLEGE

If your school offers Advanced Placement courses, consider taking biology, chemistry, and physics. These courses are not a requirement for CSD programs, but you will be surprised to find that undergraduate and graduate communication sciences courses reintroduce some of the concepts you learn in these courses. With all that you will be learning in your undergraduate coursework, having a good background in science will certainly be an advantage to you.

## TAKE WRITING COURSES

You will use your writing skills frequently during your undergraduate and graduate coursework, so focusing on developing these skills will pay off when you write term papers, observation reports, and, possibly, a thesis. Having excellent writing skills is also helpful when writing essays for scholarships and admittance into academic programs. Any course that strengthens your writing skills will be extremely useful. Find out if your high school offers a rhetoric or an advanced grammar course and take it if possible. Make it easier on yourself by becoming a good writer now. Try to think like an English teacher when you write. Make a list of feedback that your teacher gives on your English papers so that you learn from your mistakes, such as using active voice instead of passive voice. The more you write, the easier the process will become and the more proficient you will be. Take advantage of any opportunity you have to practice your writing skills and to get constructive feedback on your work.

## FIND A COLLEGE/UNIVERSITY OFFERING A MAJOR IN COMMUNICATION SCIENCES AND DISORDERS

Not all universities and colleges have a CSD program. On university or college Web sites, search with keywords such as "audiology," "speech–language pathology," and "communication disorders." Depending on the program, the department may be called *communication disorders and sciences, communication disorders,* or *communicative disorders.* For a list of colleges and universities that offer CSD programs, you can also access the Web sites of Council of Academic Programs in Communication Sciences and Disorders (CAPCSD) and the National Academy of Preprofessional Programs in Communication Sciences and Disorders (NAPP).

## VISIT A NATIONAL STUDENT SPEECH LANGUAGE HEARING ASSOCIATION CHAPTER

To learn more about undergraduate coursework in CSD and to talk with students about their experience, visit a local college or university chapter of the NSSLHA. To find a chapter in your state, go to the Chapters section of the NSSLHA Web site and click the link "Find a NSSLHA Chapter in your area." Call the university's CSD department (which may also be called *communication disorders and sciences* or *communicative disorders*) and ask for the NSSLHA chapter advisor or a department volunteer. Explain to the chapter advisor, or the department volunteer, that you are a high school student and that, with permission, you would like to attend the next NSSLHA meeting. Ask for the date, time, and location of the meeting. Then ask for the chapter president's e-mail address. Let the chapter advisor know that you would like to talk with the president about the department after the meeting. Go prepared with questions, a pen, and a notebook. Make sure that you thank the chapter president or any other students for taking the time to meet with you. It would be a good idea to also send a thank-you note to let them know you appreciate their help.

## VISIT THE COMMUNICATION SCIENCES AND DISORDERS DEPARTMENT WHERE YOU ARE APPLYING TO COLLEGE

Visiting the colleges and universities, and their CSD departments, you are applying to is an excellent way to determine whether the campus is the right fit for you. When you are researching the institution, search the department Web site for the department telephone number. Then call and speak to an undergraduate advisor or his or her secretary. Make an appointment to discuss the program on the day of your visit. Explain that you are a high school student.

During the appointment, you may want to ask the advisor:

- What are the prerequisites for entering the program?
- Is there an application process to enter the undergraduate major? May I have the application?
- What is the minimum GPA requirement?
- Do you have a list of courses for undergraduates?

- Is there an active NSSLHA chapter? What types of activities does the chapter do?
- Is there a graduate program for audiology and speech–language pathology?
- What percentage of your students who apply for graduate school in audiology or speech–language pathology get into a program?

## ORDER A COMPLIMENTARY SUBSCRIPTION TO NSSLHA'S NEWSLETTER

It is not too soon to start learning about the academic and professional issues CSD majors face. The NSSLHA newsletter, *NSSLHA Now*, is an excellent resource to find out more about CSD students and developments in CSD programs and the professions. Visit the NSSLHA Web site and use the Publications section to get a complimentary subscription to *NSSLHA Now.*

## GET INVOLVED

By getting involved in clubs, groups, or teams, you will learn more about yourself and other people, and be more knowledgeable about a variety of topics. Getting involved can help you develop good interpersonal skills and self-confidence, which are important for a successful career in CSD. Depending on your interests and what is available at your high school or in your community, you may want to consider getting involved with the student newspaper, drama club, band, yearbook, prayer group, student council, track team, other team sports, and so on. Besides being a great way to meet people and enjoy great experiences, colleges usually like students to be well rounded. Plus, having a variety of experiences may make it easier to relate to your clients and their families. Clients usually brighten up when clinicians have experience in an activity that the clients currently, or used to, do, such as sports or hobbies. Moreover, when you decide to work with children, having many different experiences of your own to draw upon could be very helpful in putting them at ease and making them feel comfortable with you.

## CONSIDER WORKING PART-TIME

Working while in high school may or may not be the best option for you. Calculate how many hours of homework you have each night, average sleep that you need to feel alert, and the time you devote for extracurricular activities, such as band, cross-country practice, speech club, and drama. Also consider whether you have easy access to transportation (e.g., car or bike). Speak with your parents/guardians about how they feel about you working. If you decide to work, find a part-time job that will give you experience related to CSD. Apply to be a day-camp counselor for children with special needs, childcare worker, nursing home worker, summer time teacher's aide of special needs, tutor, and so on. Any experience you gain can be useful down the road in helping you understand material in your classes, even applying to graduate school, and working with clients.

## VOLUNTEER

Consider volunteering at a hospital if the medical setting interests you. Volunteering at a hospital is a great way to learn about the medical professions. You can request to volunteer in the hearing; ear, nose, and throat; or speech–language pathology clinics. Volunteering in the emergency room, admitting, birthing floor, and other areas of the hospital will give you a great insight into how a hospital functions. You will draw on these experiences when you are taking undergraduate and graduate courses in CSD. Volunteering can also be an excellent way to start thinking about any work settings you may one day consider.

## CONCLUSION

High school students seem to be getting busier and busier all the time. With schoolwork, extracurriculars, part-time jobs, spending time with friends, and the stress of applying to college, you may feel like you do not have any time left to spend planning for a career that seems so far off. Reading through this chapter, though, should help you realize that there are many things you can start doing now that will have a positive impact down the road. Some of these suggestions, such as taking science and writing classes, are good ideas regardless of what major you decide to pursue. Other suggestions, such as job shadowing, may require a little more effort. On the one hand, learning early on that you are interested in pursuing a particular degree can give you the advantage in a sometimes competitive college application process. On the other hand, learning early about what you really *do not* want to do for a living can save you a lot of hassle later on (such as finding yourself behind in credits once you change majors, or needing to change colleges because the path you thought you wanted to pursue turns out to be not for you).

# CHAPTER 5

# Advice for Freshman and Sophomore Years

## INTRODUCTION

The first two years of college are the foundation of your academic career. In your freshman year, you will likely take university-wide courses that are required for graduation (e.g., biology, writing, calculus, anthropology). By sophomore year, you are likely to take at least a few courses in or related to your major (e.g., introduction to communication sciences and disorders [CSD], introduction to linguistics). No matter how exciting the freshman year may seem, the transition from high school to college can be daunting. The keys to conquering the freshman and sophomore years are following good academic advice and balancing a social life and school life.

Choosing your required courses can be confusing. Fortunately, every student has an academic advisor. Get to know your academic advisor because he or she will help you navigate through the required courses and can offer advice on selecting any electives toward your major (if that is an option during your freshman year).

As you continue through your studies, make sure you make time for yourself. Students in CSD tend to overwork themselves. If you find yourself overworking, try having fun with friends at least once a week. Relaxation and laughter are good for you—so is achieving balance between your academic, social, and personal commitments. When you take time off, you feel refreshed and ready to taken on your assignments.

This chapter provides advice on achieving success through your freshman and sophomore years, using ways beyond your regular coursework so that you become even more involved in your future profession. Keep track of your progress using the checklist in Figure 5-1.

## JOIN YOUR CAMPUS CHAPTER OF NATIONAL STUDENT SPEECH LANGUAGE HEARING ASSOCIATION

As a freshman, you will find that there are many organizations, groups, and clubs that are looking forward to your involvement. Consider becoming an active member of your local National Student Speech Language Hearing Association (NSSLHA) chapter. Being involved with NSSLHA will give you opportunities

- [ ] Join your campus chapter of NSSLHA
- [ ] Join NSSLHA
- [ ] Make a timeline of your courses from now until graduation
- [ ] Focus on your GPA
- [ ] Make your face and name known
- [ ] Find out if your university has an undergraduate research program
- [ ] Observe speech and/or hearing therapy
- [ ] Save your textbooks and notes
- [ ] Create a résumé
- [ ] Download a graduate school application
- [ ] Keep a college contact list
- [ ] Apply for student membership in your state's speech-language-hearing association
- [ ] Start exploring a specific discipline or professional area of interest
- [ ] Consider taking a foreign language or sign language class
- [ ] Consider taking a class on cultural diversity
- [ ] Consider getting a minor
- [ ] Take care of any teaching certification requirements as an undergraduate

**Figure 5-1**  Checklist for freshman and sophomore years *(Source: Delmar/Cengage Learning.)*

to interact with people who are in your major as well as opportunities to get involved with issues that concern your future profession.

You may volunteer for a committee. Building relationships and staying involved in your department is the best way to access resources that will help you throughout your academic career. Moreover, joining a committee to solve a problem, planning an event, and achieving a goal are a great way to network and have fun. Also consider running for an office in your local NSSLHA chapter, so you can gain leadership experience, which will be of interest to future employers.

## JOIN NATIONAL STUDENT SPEECH LANGUAGE HEARING ASSOCIATION

In addition to your local NSSLHA chapter, you may want to join the national organization. (For more information on the benefits of joining NSSLHA, see Chapter 24, or visit the NSSLHA Web site.) As a national member, you have access to online journals, discounts on products and services, among others. To maintain your national membership benefits, remember to renew your membership annually.

Many people are not aware that NSSLHA is a student-run membership association. As a member of the national association, you are represented by 1 of 11 students. Communicate with your regional councilor (RC) to gather more information. A list of RCs and their contact information are available on the NSSLHA Web site.

## MAKE A TIMELINE OF YOUR COURSES FROM NOW UNTIL GRADUATION

The number of courses that you need to take before you graduate may overwhelm you. Keep yourself organized by making a timeline of all your courses from your first year through graduation. To have the right course information, make an appointment with your academic advisor to plan out your coursework. The outline will ensure that you avoid taking unnecessary courses and that you choose elective courses of your interest.

A mix of challenging and easy courses will help you maintain a healthy and manageable academic course load. Of note, however, not all universities allow you to choose your courses.

## FOCUS ON YOUR GRADE POINT AVERAGE

With all the excitement surrounding the first year of college, some freshmen have a hard time staying focused on studying. Your grades determine whether you qualify for a graduate school and a scholarship. To enter most graduate schools, you need a minimum of a 3.0 grade point average (GPA) on a 4.0 scale. The most competitive schools, however, accept only students who have at least a 3.5 GPA. What if your GPA is not where you need it to be? Most campuses have numerous resources available to help you achieve academic success. There are writing centers and tutors who can help you, as well as professor office hours. If you find yourself falling behind or having trouble adjusting to college-level work, seek appropriate help.

Having strong study skills, along with time management skills, will make a tremendous difference as you move on through your undergraduate studies into graduate school! Therefore, it is a good idea to take a time management course and a study skills course.

## MAKE YOUR NAME AND FACE KNOWN

Make your presence felt in the department and let professors get to know you. For example, be actively involved in your local NSSLHA chapter or volunteer whenever the department needs help with something. This approach allows them to watch you grow through your college career. Consequently, when you have a class with these professors, you will feel more comfortable approaching them with questions. Also, when applying for graduate school, these professors will be able to write you powerful letters of recommendation. *Don't be just a number!*

If you do not understand something or want to learn more about a topic, meet with your professors during their office hours. Do not hesitate to e-mail your professor, stay after class, and seek help if you need one. Universities pay professors to teach you the concepts and answer your questions. Get your money's worth! Most professors prefer students who are inquisitive and want to learn. Make use of your professors' office hours so they have the opportunity to get to know you as a student.

## FIND OUT IF YOUR UNIVERSITY HAS AN UNDERGRADUATE RESEARCH PROGRAM

Research programs teach research procedures to students by pairing them with a researcher in their area of interest, enabling them to learn how research is conducted and become knowledgeable about a specific topic. Contact your CSD department chairperson or a CSD professor to determine whether such an opportunity is available to you. If your college does not have a specific program (usually only larger universities have such programs), contact the head of your department and ask if you can assist a professor in the department with research. A program may not be in place, but there are professors in need of research assistance. At many universities, you can earn academic credit by registering the experience as an independent study. Research experience also looks great on résumés when applying to graduate school!

Another advantage of a research program is the opportunity to learn the American Psychological Association (APA) style manual, *Publication Manual of the American Psychological Association.* Many freshman English classes require students to use the *MLA Handbook for Writers of Research Papers* when writing papers. In CSD, however, students use the APA style manual to write papers. If you are given a choice between Modern Language Association (MLA) and APA style of documentation, practice using APA. To learn how to properly format and document references, purchase an APA book from a local bookstore or go to the APA Web site).

## OBSERVE SPEECH AND/OR HEARING THERAPY

Observation at a campus CSD clinic is a great way to learn about clinical practice and the profession. As a freshman, any observations you do are separate from American Speech–Language–Hearing Association (ASHA's) required observation hours. You will learn more about these required hours during your junior or senior years. To observe, first find out whether your campus has a CSD clinic and then contact the clinic director or coordinator. If there are opportunities to observe, make sure that you ask about the clinic and follow any procedures required at the clinic, such as signing in, following a particular dress code, and ways to interact with clients.

To learn more about professionals working outside an academic setting, you can observe an audiologist or a speech–language pathologist (SLP) working in a hospital, school, or private practice. You can locate potential individuals to observe by looking through the telephone book or speaking with professors or individuals associated with your campus clinic. Again, these hours are to help you learn more about the profession and are separate from ASHA's required observation hours; however, if a course at the undergraduate level requires observation hours, these may be able to count toward that requirement. If possible, try to complete 10–15 hours of observations by the end of the school year. Observing now will help make the discussions in your future courses much more concrete (which may consequently make the material easier to learn). Come with questions for the audiologist or SLP.

Use the summer as an opportunity to volunteer at a clinic or a hospital or apply for a summer job related to CSD. If you do not know where to look for these opportunities, ask your NSSLHA advisor or academic program director. Or you may visit the ASHA online Career Center on the ASHA Web site for a list of professionals in your area. Building good relationships with a clinic or hospital now may mean future volunteer opportunities, or even employment opportunities down the line. Be sure to include all volunteer experiences on your résumé.

## SAVE YOUR TEXTBOOKS AND NOTES

Students often look to the end of the semester as an opportunity to sell back books and make a little extra money. How disappointing it can be, though, when that text you originally paid $80.00 for, and sold back for $10.00, turns out to be a resource you wish you had for a graduate course. As you start taking courses that relate to your major, you will find it helpful to save your textbooks. Not only might they be required in another class, but they can be excellent resources and references for papers and projects (even in graduate school and professional practice). It is also a good idea to save your notes as references (e.g., psychology, education, and statistics notes).

Use 3-ring binders to organize your notes, with tabs to separate subjects. To make it easier to find your notes, write down all of the materials in the binder on two labels. Attach one sticky label to the spine of the binder, and the other to the front of the binder. The end of the semester is a good time to put your note binder together because the material is still fresh in your mind. Appendix A provides a complete list of items to help you get organized.

When you are in graduate school, you will be grateful that you have been organized since freshman year. To become a nationally certified clinician after graduate school, you will be required to take a comprehensive examination that covers all of the material from your undergraduate major and graduate coursework. It will make preparation for this examination a lot less stressful if you have that binder for reference. Furthermore, these textbooks and notes are the foundation of your professional library.

# CREATE A RÉSUMÉ
. . . . . . . . . . . . . . . . . . . . . .

A résumé is a document that tells a prospective employer about your professional experience, education, and interests. Although you may not have much professional experience, it is a good idea to keep track of all the different jobs and positions you hold. Record all your work experiences, volunteer services, and educational experiences in a working résumé. If your campus has a career center, you can make an appointment to learn how to write a résumé. If your campus does not have a career center, ask a librarian to help you find a book about writing résumés. Starting a résumé now will help you realize what you need to accomplish over the next few years. Furthermore, a résumé will be useful when you are applying to honor societies, undergraduate programs (if applicable), graduate programs, jobs, and scholarships. For more information on drafting a résumé, see Chapter 23.

## DOWNLOAD A GRADUATE SCHOOL APPLICATION
. . . . . . . . . . . . . . . . . . . . . . . . . . . . . . . . . . . . . . . . . . . . . . . . . . .

If graduate school is a possibility, start looking at graduate school applications, in preparation for what you will need to do when you are ready to apply. Go to the Internet and download an application form from your "dream school" or CSD program. Look over the application now, and you can spend the next few years making sure that you have enough experiences to fill in the application as an ideal candidate. Before you know it, your dream school may become a reality.

It is also important to speak with a graduate student in a CSD program. Graduate students are very knowledgeable and may be more approachable than some professors are. They can let you know what to expect after graduating with your bachelor's degree. If your school only has an undergraduate program, contact your NSSLHA RC to find a graduate student in your region who can answer your questions and give advice.

## KEEP A COLLEGE CONTACT LIST
. . . . . . . . . . . . . . . . . . . . . . . . . . . . . . . . . . . .

The college contact worksheet in Figure 5-2 is an excellent resource for keeping track of important names, numbers, and addresses. Updating this list every

**Name of University Academic Advisor**_____

Address _____

Telephone Number _____

E-mail _____

*(continues)*

**Figure 5-2** College contact worksheet

**Name of CSD Academic Advisor** _____

Address _____

Telephone Number _____

E-mail _____

**Name of NSSLHA Advisor** _____

Address _____

Telephone Number _____

E-mail _____

**Name of NSSLHA Chapter President** _____

Address _____

Telephone Number _____

E-mail _____

**Name of NSSLHA Regional Councilor** _____

Address _____

Telephone Number _____

E-mail _____

**Name of Mentor** _____

Address _____

Telephone Number _____

E-mail _____

**Name of Professor Who Can Write You a Letter of Recommendation** _____

Address _____

Telephone Number _____

E-mail _____

**Figure 5-2** (_Continued_)

**Name of State Association** _____

Address _____

Telephone Number _____

E-mail _____


**Other** _____

Telephone Number _____

Web Site _____

E-mail _____

You can update this form every academic school year to assist you when visiting programs, completing grants and scholarship applications, completing college applications, or just to keep track of people in the profession with whom you come into contact.

**Figure 5-2** (*Continued*)

academic school year will enable you to contact key individuals when you have questions. This list will also make it easier when you fill out scholarship and graduate school applications. Some people you might want to include in this list are professionals you observed and your professors.

## APPLY FOR STUDENT MEMBERSHIP IN YOUR STATE'S SPEECH–LANGUAGE–HEARING ASSOCIATION

All 50 states and the District of Columbia have state speech–language–hearing associations that oversee regulatory policy and licensure of audiologists and SLPs. Most state speech–language–hearing associations allow students to become members at a reduced fee. To verify that you are a student, the state associations may ask, on your applications, for a signature from the head of your department. State associations usually have newsletters and conferences that provide information beyond what is taught in the classroom. Visit the ASHA Web site to locate the state association in your area. Figure 5-3 provides a list of reasons why students should join a state association.

Become an active student member of your state association and volunteer at a state association convention. State associations are always on the lookout for volunteers to help at registration desks, help with stuffing envelopes, and

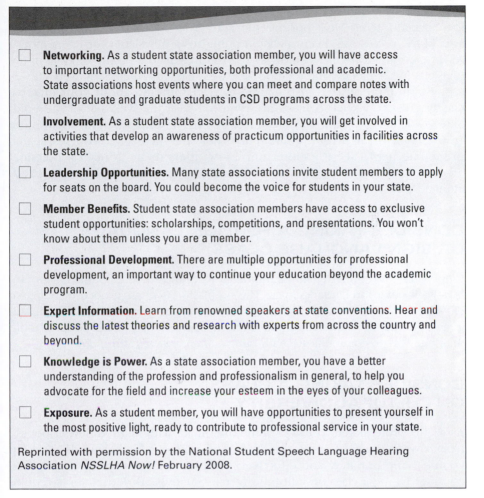

☐ **Networking.** As a student state association member, you will have access to important networking opportunities, both professional and academic. State associations host events where you can meet and compare notes with undergraduate and graduate students in CSD programs across the state.

☐ **Involvement.** As a student state association member, you will get involved in activities that develop an awareness of practicum opportunities in facilities across the state.

☐ **Leadership Opportunities.** Many state associations invite student members to apply for seats on the board. You could become the voice for students in your state.

☐ **Member Benefits.** Student state association members have access to exclusive student opportunities: scholarships, competitions, and presentations. You won't know about them unless you are a member.

☐ **Professional Development.** There are multiple opportunities for professional development, an important way to continue your education beyond the academic program.

☐ **Expert Information.** Learn from renowned speakers at state conventions. Hear and discuss the latest theories and research with experts from across the country and beyond.

☐ **Knowledge is Power.** As a state association member, you have a better understanding of the profession and professionalism in general, to help you advocate for the field and increase your esteem in the eyes of your colleagues.

☐ **Exposure.** As a student member, you will have opportunities to present yourself in the most positive light, ready to contribute to professional service in your state.

Reprinted with permission by the National Student Speech Language Hearing Association *NSSLHA Now!* February 2008.

**Figure 5-3** Why join a state association?

take care of paperwork. Call your state association to ask whom to contact to volunteer at the convention. When you are not volunteering at the convention, you can attend educational sessions. Remember to add the volunteer experience and your educational sessions to your résumé!

## START EXPLORING A SPECIFIC DISCIPLINE OR PROFESSIONAL AREA OF INTEREST

It is never too early to start preparing for graduate school. Use this time to start asking more questions about what really interests you in CSD and start finding educational and volunteer opportunities in that area of interest. Let your program's faculty and the resources available from national and local NSSLHA assist you in identifying your interests.

NSSLHA members can join ASHA's Special Interest Divisions at a reduced fee. Special Interest Divisions are specialty groups that focus on a particular area of the profession. Every division publishes a newsletter for its members. ASHA currently recognizes 16 divisions. You may read a profile of each of the divisions in Chapter 26. Information is also available on the ASHA Web site.

Sophomore year is also a time to start thinking about your elective classes. To know what courses are required, visit the Web site of the graduate-level CSD program you are interested in. If your program offers these courses, take them. If your program does not offer the needed courses, search in the Internet to see if another university offers them. Contact a potential graduate program and see if the credit would transfer. Use your undergraduate time wisely.

## CONSIDER TAKING A FOREIGN LANGUAGE OR SIGN LANGUAGE CLASS

Employers often prefer to hire candidates who know some Spanish, sign language, or other foreign languages. The profession is in great need of bilingual clinicians. You will be very marketable when you graduate with a foreign language. No matter what setting you work in, you will be grateful to have more than one way to communicate with others. *Make yourself stand out!*

## CONSIDER TAKING A CLASS ON CULTURAL DIVERSITY

As a CSD professional, you will come in contact with many different people from a wide range of cultural, ethnic, and religious backgrounds. To help you deal appropriately and effectively with these clients and their families, consider taking a class on cultural diversity. Many CSD departments require these courses; however, taking a course on cultural diversity through another department will also prove to be very valuable. For additional suggestions, see Chapter 16.

## CONSIDER GETTING A MINOR

Some students have a minor, but it is not a requirement in the field. Sometimes, there is not enough time or financial means to earn a minor and graduate in four years. However, if there is an area of interest that you would like to pursue, then go for it! Sign language, psychology, special education, elementary education, family studies, statistics, linguistics, gerontology, communications, and Spanish are some common minors that students in CSD programs consider. If you are interested in pursuing a minor, make sure that you speak with your academic advisor to map out the courses you should be taking in each semester. However, ensure that you do not make a mistake that may delay your date of graduation.

# TAKE CARE OF ANY TEACHING CERTIFICATION REQUIREMENTS AS AN UNDERGRADUATE

If you are interested in working in a school setting, make sure you are aware of the requirements. In fact, some states require you to have a teaching certificate to work in a hospital because you could work with children from schools that do not have an audiologist or have a shortage of SLPs. Most states require professionals to take certain special education coursework and have teaching experience. To learn more about teaching certification requirements, contact your academic advisor, NSSLHA chapter advisor, state board of education, and an audiologist or an SLP who works in a school.

Even if you do not wish to work in a school setting, getting your certification gives you additional options for future employment. These classes will strengthen your teaching skills and will give you the opportunity to interact with other future professionals, such as special education teachers, general education teachers, occupational therapists, and physical therapists. Collaborating with others is an important skill to learn, especially when you work on interdisciplinary teams for the benefit of your future clients.

Start thinking about research questions that you might want to address in a thesis. A thesis is a major project investigating a particular question. If you are interested in earning doctorate, a thesis will help you decide whether you enjoy the research process. It is helpful to keep a notebook of possible research questions and ideas. As you are researching projects for class or listening to lectures, write down any questions or thoughts that come to mind that you may want to research further. This notebook will be invaluable when you begin to formulate your thesis!

## CONCLUSION

In freshman and sophomore years, many new experiences and learning opportunities are open to you. Enjoy this time but also stay focused on your long-term goal: to work as a CSD professional. Although your career as a practicing audiologist, SLP, or speech–language–hearing scientist may be a long way off, by using the suggestions in this chapter you can gain valuable experiences that will follow you through your education into your professional career.

# CHAPTER 6

# Advice for Junior and Senior Years

## INTRODUCTION

Your junior and senior years of college can be very exciting. These are the years that you will probably take most of your communication sciences and disorders (CSD) courses. You now face important decisions about what direction to take after graduation. In addition to all these important decisions (e.g., where to apply to graduate school, how to pay for more education), you still have a rigorous year of coursework ahead. Junior and senior years can be very demanding, as well. Your academic courses become more in depth, and your get more involved in your homework and projects. Moreover, you will be spending time preparing for the Graduate Record Examination (GRE) and investigating and applying for graduate schools—all while you continue to build your résumé. This chapter provides tips on making the most of your junior and senior years of college. Use the checklist in Figure 6-1 to keep track of your progress.

☐ Remain focused on your GPA

☐ Find out if you can participate in a directed study

☐ Attend the ASHA convention in November

☐ Attend and volunteer at your state association convention

☐ Apply for a regional councilor position in NSSLHA

☐ Start researching CSD graduate programs

☐ Take the GRE early

☐ Update your résumé

☐ Ask about an assistantship position

☐ Apply for financial aid and other scholarship programs in late fall or early winter

☐ Keep track of all deadlines for applications

☐ If accepted to several graduate programs, decide which you want to attend

☐ Consider taking time off before entering a graduate program

**Figure 6-1** Checklist for junior and senior years *(Source: Delmar/Cengage Learning.)*

# REMAIN FOCUSED ON YOUR GRADE POINT AVERAGE

As you move from the general and introductory courses to more specialized topics in your major, you may find the material more interesting, but more challenging as well. With the decision to apply to graduate school around the corner, it is more important than ever to maintain your grade point average (GPA) to make yourself a competitive candidate. As mentioned in Chapter 5, most graduate schools require a minimum of 3.0 GPA, with some schools requiring a minimum of 3.5 GPA. If you believe you need help, make use of the resources available on campus, and find a graduate student who can tutor you, or work with your professors during their office hours.

# FIND OUT IF YOU CAN PARTICIPATE IN A DIRECTED STUDY

A directed study is an opportunity for a student to work on a research project with a professor, with a common research interest. You may work alongside a professor for a semester, in a clinic or laboratory, while earning academic credit. If your program does not already have a directed study environment in place, introduce the concept to your department. This approach is a great way to get your research career started with a mentor who you trust to guide you through the process. This experience will be useful when applying for research-related positions as a graduate student; professors usually like to hire students who have research experience.

# ATTEND THE AMERICAN SPEECH–LANGUAGE–HEARING ASSOCIATION CONVENTION IN NOVEMBER

The further along you get in your studies, the more you will benefit from attending the American Speech–Language–Hearing Association (ASHA) convention. If you cannot afford to attend, consider applying to volunteer at the ASHA convention. Students who volunteer at the convention get their registration paid, but you can only be selected as a volunteer one time. If you have applied in the past, but you were not accepted, by all means, apply again. For more information on the ASHA convention, see Chapter 25.

# ATTEND AND VOLUNTEER AT YOUR STATE ASSOCIATION CONVENTION

Although the ASHA convention is a fantastic place to attend sessions and be exposed to hot topics of interest in the profession, your state convention offers informative sessions and access to vendors and resources, is less expensive, and is usually closer than the national convention. Presenters and sessions are always changing, so if you have attended the state convention in the past, be sure to attend again. Now that you have taken multiple courses in your program, the sessions will reinforce what you have been learning. If you have not previously attended a convention, commit to going during your junior and years. This is an excellent way of networking with students and professionals and may lead to professional opportunities as a student.

# APPLY FOR A REGIONAL COUNCILOR POSITION IN NATIONAL STUDENT SPEECH LANGUAGE HEARING ASSOCIATION

Getting involved at the national level of National Student Speech Language Hearing Association (NSSLHA) will give you the opportunity to meet future CSD leaders, as well as make contact with leaders of ASHA. A regional councilor (RC) acts as a liaison between the NSSLHA executive council and the local NSSLHA chapters within the region. The RC regularly communicates with NSSLHA chapters, attends biannual executive council meetings, and sits on an ASHA board or committee. NSSLHA accepts applications for RC every February, and they are available on the NSSLHA Web site.

# START RESEARCHING COMMUNICATION SCIENCES AND DISORDERS GRADUATE PROGRAMS

By your junior year, you should have an idea of whether you want to pursue a graduate degree in communication sciences. During your junior year, you should start researching graduate programs that are of interest to you. You might start your research at the Graduate School Fair hosted by NSSLHA during the ASHA convention. Here, students can gather information about the different graduate programs available and can meet with faculty from many of the schools.

As you are considering different programs, remember that to become an ASHA-certified audiologist or speech–language pathologist (SLP), you must complete graduate coursework from a program accredited by the Council on Academic Accreditation in Audiology and Speech–Language Pathology (CAA) of the ASHA. If you are not able to make it to the Graduate School Fair, there is another option for researching graduate programs, EdFind! EdFind is ASHA's online, on-demand academic program search engine to identify graduate programs accredited by the CAA. EdFind is easily accessible on the ASHA Web site.

As you begin looking for a graduate program, keep an open mind. Look at many different schools across the country—the right program for you and your academic interests could be across the street or across the country, but you will never know if you do not thoroughly investigate your options. Figure 6-2 provides tips for selecting a graduate program.

**Admission Criteria.** Do you make the grade? Review the criteria stated on the department's Web site. Make sure that you meet at least the minimal standards for admission. Many programs require this before they will even consider your application.

**Financial Support.** Are there opportunities to defray the costs of graduate school? Remember that there may be opportunities both inside and outside the department. Ask about funding through grants as well as additional graduate funding through other departments on campus.

**Scope of Faculty Specialization.** Will I be adequately trained in the scope of practice? As you prepare to practice as an audiologist or speech-language pathologist, make sure you will be well trained in every facet of the profession. A strong program will have faculty that specialize in topics across the scope of practice. You want to be prepared for anything.

**Full-Time/Part-Time Student Ratio.** Is there flexibility, such as distance learning and part-time programming? Today's graduate student pool includes many who fit in the "nontraditional" category. If that describes you, be sure to ask about individual and nontraditional programming.

**Strengths of the Academic Program.** Are there particularly strong faculty in my areas of interest? Faculty with parallel interests may provide you with important opportunities to further develop your interest and hone your skills.

**Research.** Is there training and opportunity to develop research interests? Research is the backbone of our profession; it guides both our knowledge and practice. You want a program that can train you to be a critical consumer of research.

**Strengths of the Clinical Education Program.** Are there adequate training opportunities with a range of both on-site and off-site experiences? To be prepared for the scope of practice that exists across the life span, you want training opportunities that reflect a variety of populations.

**Practicum Experience.** Is assistance available for externship placements? As you prepare for your final training experiences, the possibilities may seem endless. You will want to inquire about assistance in making contact with facilities, establishing contracts, obtaining insurance, and so on.

*(continues)*

**Figure 6-2** Tips for selecting a graduate program

**Uniqueness.** What features of the program make it stand out? This is your chosen life career. Pick the program with outstanding features that seem tailor-made for you.

**The School's NSSLHA Chapter.** You want to choose a program that will allow you continued professional development through an active NSSLHA chapter. This experience will prepare you for an active role in the professional association, ASHA.

Reprinted with permission by the National Student Speech Language Hearing Association *NSSLHA Now!* November 2005

**Figure 6-2** *(Continued)*

## TAKE THE GRADUATE RECORD EXAMINATION EARLY

The GRE is the entrance examination required for most graduate-level programs. Universities often use these scores to nominate students for fellowships, which can pay a student's tuition fees and provide a stipend. The average GRE acceptance score for a graduate CSD program is probably higher than the overall university-required score.

Make sure you know the scores that you will need for acceptance into the programs you are interested in and what scores are needed to be competitive for fellowships (which often require high GRE scores). If your scores are at or above the minimum to get into a program and your other areas of application are strong (e.g. GPA, letters of recommendation, volunteer experience, and essays), then you may not need to pay thousands of dollars to get superior GRE scores.

You will want to start studying for the GRE during the end of your junior year. Create a study plan that works best for you. To help direct your studying and to take practice tests, you may want to purchase a review book with a CD-ROM. To save money, find out whether a library on your campus has GRE review books.

Another way to prepare for the GRE is with a review course. Ask your academic advisor or office of student affairs whether your university is offering any GRE courses. Also, inquire about review courses through a learning center or a professional test-taking service in your area. However, these courses can cost from $400 to $2,000. Plan accordingly if you choose to take a review course. Instead of a formal course, some review agencies offer online courses that are in the $100 to $300 range. An online course allows you to work at your own pace. Check with the review agencies for exact prices. Before committing a significant amount of money to a review course, take a practice examination in a GRE review book to get a sense of how much preparation you may need.

Consider enrolling in a basic algebra course at your local community college the summer prior to your senior year. If you have not taken a mathematics course in several years, a basic algebra course will act as a good review of mathematics concepts that are easy to forget without frequent use. Courses at a community college are often less expensive than university courses, and summer classes offer flexible options for class length, format, and time of day to better fit with your schedule.

Do not wait until the last minute to take the GRE. Sign up for a summer or early fall examination time. By taking the GRE in the summer, you can focus on studying for the GRE while not having to worry about coursework at the same time. Taking the GRE early makes it possible for you to raise your scores if necessary because you have time to retake the examination before application deadlines arrive. Moreover, if you do well the first time, you will not need to worry about the GRE ever again. However, if you have to take the examination more than once, it is perfectly okay. Many students aspire to have high scores on the GRE and retest several times. Visit the GRE Web site for registration information.

Do not get discouraged by the GRE examination—it can be a difficult examination, but your score will not necessarily make or break your chances of getting into graduate school. To know how much GRE scores are emphasized when reviewing applications, speak with the academic program's department chair or advisor where you are planning to apply. GRE scores are a piece of the admissions process, but remember the GPA you have worked hard to maintain, volunteer and/or paid work, your essay, and all the other great things you have listed on your résumé will be looked at carefully by the admissions board.

## UPDATE YOUR RÉSUMÉ

If you have been following the advice for the freshman and sophomore in Chapter 5, you should have started your résumé. If you have not started writing your résumé, now is a good time to start. For more information on updating résumés, read Chapter 23.

## ASK ABOUT AN ASSISTANTSHIP POSITION

Research, teaching, clinical, and project assistantships are some of the assistantships available in graduate audiology and speech–language pathology programs. Some assistantships offer students a tuition waiver and/or stipend if they agree to assist a professor for a fixed number of hours per week (e.g., 15–20 hours). Most schools have a limited number of assistantships, so apply early and often. Assistantship opportunities may vary throughout the year. For instance, a professor may look for a research assistant after receiving a grant during the middle of an academic year. Contact a professor with whom you would like to work, let him or her know that you would be interested in an assistantship position, and stay in regular contact with that person if he or she indicates there may be something available later in the year.

## APPLY FOR FINANCIAL AID AND OTHER SCHOLARSHIP PROGRAMS IN LATE FALL OR EARLY WINTER

Once you have decided what school you will attend, create a budget for yourself. Also consider the cost of rent, bills (e.g., electric, water, heat, telephone, cell phone, Internet access), food, car payments, car insurance, books and new equipment (e.g., otoscope), furniture, clothing, and travel to visit family and friends. Plan how many hours you will work during graduate school. Talk to current graduate students and find out how many hours per week is realistically manageable.

Realize that not all graduate students work and you should take into account the stress involved in having a job. Some students work too many hours per week, and they miss out on learning much of the information they are paying to learn. Try to keep a healthy balance between school and what you may need to do to pay for school.

Although graduate school can be a considerable financial commitment, there are many great options for helping fund this stage of your education. Graduate assistantships, loans, and grants are often available, depending on the school you plan to attend and on your particular situation. For more information on applying for financial aid and scholarships, see Chapter 19.

## KEEP TRACK OF ALL DEADLINES FOR APPLICATIONS

For fall admissions, some programs have deadlines as early as December 1. Make sure that you mail all of the information to the right departments well before the deadlines. After you mail your applications, you will need to call each school's CSD department to make sure it received all of the proper information. Sometimes, letters of recommendation are lost or GRE scores are filed in the wrong place. Do not assume the departments received all of your information. Because most programs have many applicants, they will not contact you if they are missing part of your application. They simply will not review your application. Continue to call until you have verification that your application is complete. Use the graduate school application worksheet in Figure 6-3 to keep track of your graduate school applications and the graduate school recommendation sheet in Figure 6-4 to track letters of recommendation. As a reminder, be sure to send a thank-you note to anyone who wrote a letter of recommendation for you.

**Name of Institution:** _____

Web Site for Program: _____

Web Site for Online Application: _____

Username for Online Application: _____

Password for Online Application: _____

Application Fee: _____

Address for Application Fee If Not Paid Online: _____

Address to Send Letters of Reference: _____

Address to Send Other Materials (and list specific materials): _____

Number of Letters of Reference Required: _____

Essay Prompt(s) and Page Length Requirements: _____

Due Date: _____

Date Sent: _____

Phone Number: _____

Other: _____


**Name of Institution:** _____

Web Site for Program: _____

Web Site for Online Application: _____

Username for Online Application: _____

Password for Online Application: _____

Application Fee: _____

Address for Application Fee If Not Paid Online: _____

Address to Send Letters of Reference: _____

Address to Send Other Materials (and list specific materials): _____

*(continues)*

**Figure 6-3** Graduate school application worksheet

Number of Letters of Reference Required: _____

Essay Prompt(s) and Page Length Requirements: _____

Due Date: _____

Date Sent: _____

Phone Number: _____

Other: _____

**Name of Institution:** _____

Web Site for Program: _____

Web Site for Online Application: _____

Username for Online Application: _____

Password for Online Application: _____

Application Fee: _____

Address for Application Fee If Not Paid Online: _____

Address to Send Letters of Reference: _____

Address to Send Other Materials (and list specific materials): _____

Number of Letters of Reference Required: _____

Essay Prompt(s) and Page Length Requirements: _____

Due Date: _____

Date Sent: _____

Phone Number: _____

Other: _____

**Name of Institution:** _____

Web Site for Program: _____

Web Site for Online Application: _____

Username for Online Application: _____

**Figure 6-3** (*Continued*)

Password for Online Application: _____

Application Fee: _____

Address for Application Fee If Not Paid Online: _____

Address to Send Letters of Reference: _____

Address to Send Other Materials (and list specific materials): _____

Number of Letters of Reference Required: _____

Essay Prompt(s) and Page Length Requirements: _____

Due Date: _____

Date Sent: _____

Phone Number: _____

Other: _____

This worksheet will help you organize your graduate school applications and keep track of application requirements and deadlines.

**Figure 6-3** (*Continued*)

**Professor:** _____

Title: _____

Address: _____

Phone: _____

E-mail: _____

Date Professor Prefers to Receive Packet: _____

Other: _____

*(continues)*

**Figure 6-4** Graduate school recommendation worksheet

**Professor:** _____

Title: _____

Address: _____

Phone: _____

E-mail: _____

Date Professor Prefers to Receive Packet: _____

Other: _____

**Professor:** _____

Title: _____

Address: _____

Phone: _____

E-mail: _____

Date Professor Prefers to Receive Packet: _____

Other: _____

**Former/Current Employer or Volunteer Coordinator (optional):** _____

Title: _____

Address: _____

Phone: _____

E-mail: _____

Date Employer/Volunteer Coordinator Prefers to Receive Packet: _____

Other: _____

Use this reference sheet when filling out graduate school applications to keep track of information for individuals who are writing your letters of reference.

**Figure 6-4** (*Continued*)

## IF ACCEPTED TO SEVERAL GRADUATE PROGRAMS, DECIDE WHICH YOU WANT TO ATTEND

If you get selected to more than one graduate program, making the decision on which program to attend can be daunting. The questions in Figure 6-5 are designed to help you sort through the decision-making process and to focus on those questions that will help you make the best choice for the long term.

If you have been accepted to several programs, you may have a very difficult decision before you. Ask yourself the following questions and weigh out what is most important:

- If finances were not an issue, what program would I prefer to attend?

- What program is the most affordable? What program is the most costly?

- Is the program near family or close friends? Will I know anyone at the university?

- Which cities have the highest and lowest costs of living?

- If you have a family, how does my family feel about moving to a new city?

- Is the program offering me any scholarships or tuition waivers or are there scholarship possibilities after I am in the program for a year?

- Is there good public transportation?

- What is the city like? Is there a major city within a day's driving distance? (Being in or near a major city may be nice when you need to take a break from school because most major cities have recreational events throughout the year.)

- Is there a place of worship on or near campus that I would like to attend?

- Is there one or more professors with whom I would like to do research?

- Which programs have a good academic reputation?

- Do I want a program that is more research oriented or clinically oriented? Or do I like both aspects?

*(continues)*

**Figure 6-5** Questions for choosing a graduate program *(Source: Delmar/Cengage Learning.)*

- When I called or e-mailed students in the graduate program, did they like the program? Did they seem overly stressed? Did they say that the professors are supportive and truly have an open-door policy?

- Does the program require externships that are outside the city? (Some programs require a semester where you gain clinical experience in a town that is several hours away, in a rural area.)

- How long is the program? Master's programs can last 2 or 3 years, doctoral between 5 and 7 years.

**Figure 6-5** *(Continued)*

## CONSIDER TAKING TIME OFF BEFORE ENTERING A GRADUATE PROGRAM

There are many reasons why a student may decide to take a year off before entering a graduate program, including a desire to travel, the need to work to save money, family obligations, or a feeling of being burned-out and needing some time to recharge. Whatever your personal reasons for wanting to take time off, the following are some tips for making this decision work smoothly with your plans for obtaining your graduate degree.

*Apply to Graduate Programs and (After Being Accepted) Ask If They Can Hold Your Place.* If you are early in your senior year and feel like you may need or want to take a year off before attending graduate school, keep in mind that a lot can change in a few months. Complete and submit your graduate school applications just as if you were planning on attending graduate school right after graduation. How you feel in November of your senior year could be very different from how you will feel in April—if you change your mind, you can start school in the fall and will not be forced to wait a year. If you are accepted into a program and decide that you still want to take a year off, contact the department chair, and ask if your place can be held for 1 year. You may want to offer a reason why you would like to take a year off (e.g., to earn money to pay for school, to have a child, to establish in-state residency, to take a break, for medical reasons). It depends on the situation and the program whether they will be able to hold your place, but applying to programs knowing you can try to defer admission will give you more options than simply not applying.

*Get a Job That Utilizes Your CSD Skills and Knowledge.* If you are taking a year off to earn money to pay for your graduate education, look for a position that uses the knowledge and skills gained during your CSD coursework. If you are waiting to apply to graduate programs, the experience will be helpful to your application process. Likewise, having professional experience will make the material you learn in graduate school more salient once you enter your program. Consider the following settings as you are looking for job opportunities:

- Work in a hearing and speech center or hospital.
- Work as a teacher's aid at an elementary school.
- Be a substitute teacher. In some states, you may already have completed the education requirements. Contact the state's board of education for more information.

*You Are Taking Time Off Because You Are Unsure of What Professional Direction to Take.* If you are taking a year off because you are uncertain whether you want to go into audiology or speech–language pathology, consider taking a semester of classes in another major or observing a professional in the position that interests you. Sometimes, students in CSD become interested in a related field, such as medicine, nursing, psychology, social work, special education, physical therapy, occupational therapy, or music therapy. Take time to learn about your other interests. Graduate school in audiology or speech–language pathology will be easier if you are more confident about the direction you want to go after graduation.

*Study Abroad.* If you are taking a year off from school, take the opportunity to learn about other cultures. When you are an audiologist or an SLP, you will interact with individuals from a variety of cultures. Studying abroad can assist you in having a better appreciation of different cultures and styles of communication. Furthermore, if you are interested in research, you may want to get ideas about research topics in CSD in relation to different cultures. If you go to a country that does not speak English, you can practice speaking the native language, a skill that may come in handy when you are on the job market. Moreover, studying abroad is a fun experience!

*Consider Taking Courses for Teaching Certification If You Might Work in a School Setting.* If you think you may want to work in a school setting when you have obtained your graduate degree, you may need a teaching certificate to do this, depending on where you will be working. Begin preparing for this by taking education courses during your time off. Usually, the education department offers the courses required for teaching certification. Contact an advisor at your future graduate program to see what courses you will need to take. This will lighten your load when you are a graduate student.

*Consider Completing the Requirements to Work as a Speech–Language Pathology Assistant (SLP-A).* According to the ASHA Web site, "speech-language pathology assistants are support personnel who, following academic and/or on-the-job training, perform tasks prescribed, directed, and supervised by ASHA-certified speech-language pathologists" (http://www.asha.org/about/membership-certification/faq_slpasst.htm#a1). This experience often helps students feel more confident in their clinical practicum during graduate school.

*What If You Are Not Accepted to the Program You Want to Attend?* Many graduate programs in audiology and speech–language pathology are very competitive, and there is a chance that you may not be accepted at the school you most want to attend. Consider the following options if you are faced with this situation:

- Reapply for spring admissions. However, not all programs offer spring admissions. If the program does not have spring admissions, then reapply for fall admissions of the next year.

- Contact the department of your dream school and specifically ask what you can do to be more competitive. If possible, meet with someone from the department who reviews the applications. Ask him or her to review your application with you and find out how you can make your application stronger. Plan how you will accomplish the suggestions by the next application deadline.

- Find out if you can enroll in one or two graduate courses at your dream school even though you are not in the program. You may be able to register as a "special student." However, make sure that you study smart, perform well, and get an *A* in these classes. Then, the individuals who review your application next year will see that you have the potential to succeed in their program.

- If your GPA was not competitive, retake courses in which you earned a *B* or less. At some colleges, you can retake a few courses, but there is usually a limit. Often, a university does not advertise this option, so check your university's bulletin or make an appointment with your advisor. If you cannot retake courses, take courses related to CSD (e.g., education courses) to boost your GPA (make sure that you earn *A*s).

- If your GRE scores were not competitive, take a GRE review course.

- Earn a second major in another discipline. Consider Spanish, special education, business, or marketing.

- Take a year off to work in a position related to CSD.

- If your dream school is out of state, you may be eligible for in-state residency if you work for a year. However, contact the university to learn about all the requirements for in-state residency. Check the university's Web site for phone numbers to call. Some programs try to maintain a ratio of in- and out-of-state students (usually with a higher percentage of in-state students).

## CONCLUSION

The junior and senior years are when many students really hit their stride—they feel comfortable in their school environment, understand what is expected of them, and know what to expect from their courses. Your studies should remain your primary focus, but on top of coursework, there is a lot to be done in preparation for your next step, whatever you choose it to be. Use this chapter for tips on successfully navigating the graduate school application process and to help guide your thinking as you plan for the next leg of your journey in CSD.

# Advice for the First Year of Graduate School

## INTRODUCTION

You have made it to graduate school! You are now working toward earning a Master's degree or doctorate. Students who transition from undergraduate to graduate programs soon discover that being a graduate student is much more challenging than being an undergraduate. Graduate students have to learn to think differently, write more frequently, and manage their time better.

Fortunately, during this time, faculty members do not expect you to learn everything there is to know about communication sciences and disorders (CSD). Instead, in your graduate study, you will learn the tools and techniques used to work with clients and conduct research. Once you graduate, you will fine-tune your clinical and research skills while working. This chapter offers advice for students transitioning from an undergraduate to a graduate CSD program. Use Figure 7-1 as a checklist to track your progress.

## GET READY FOR YOUR CLINICAL PRACTICUM

*Clinical practicum* (or *externship*) is clinical hours earned while a student is enrolled in the master's degree program. Audiology majors experience something similar in their second or third year of training, called *clinical rotations*. The clinical practicum is a student's first supervised experience working with clients. The time spent in the clinical practicum is *class* or *academic time*, and completing these clinical hours is a requirement for receiving your graduate degree.

For many students, the most time-consuming part of their course load is their clinical experience. Sometimes, being enrolled for only 1 credit hour of clinic can take up as much time as a 3-credit-hour graduate class. The reason is that a beginning clinician will take a lot of time to plan for sessions, gather and create materials, prepare for meetings with the clinical instructor, and write reports. With experience, student clinicians will reduce the time they spend preparing for clinics and writing reports. For more information on writing for the clinical practicum, see Chapter 22. For assistance with writing reports, see Appendix C.

☐   Get ready for your clinical practicum

☐   Get familiar with the KASA form

☐   Get organized

  ☐   Purchase a large backpack, rolling computer bag, a tote bag, and a clothes basket

  ☐   Make a timeline of your courses now until graduation

  ☐   Organize graduation-related papers in a binder

  ☐   Organize your class binders for future use

  ☐   Make daily and/or weekly lists of tasks to complete

  ☐   Constantly improve your time management skills

☐   Get help if you feel yourself getting overwhelmed

  ☐   Ask a second-year graduate student to be your mentor

  ☐   Balance your coursework and clinical work

  ☐   Take things one hour at a time

  ☐   Complete assignments early

  ☐   Be open with professors and clinical instructors when you are overwhelmed

  ☐   Take advantage of the educational opportunities offered

  ☐   You are assessed differently

  ☐   You know more than you think you know

  ☐   There can be many right answers to problems

  ☐   Relax! Most students make it through

**Figure 7-1**  Checklist for the first year of graduate school *(Source: Delmar/Cengage Learning.)*

To be a good clinician, you need to balance both coursework and clinical work. Students may fall into a routine of spending most of their time on clinical work but neglecting their traditional courses. Designate time to read your textbooks, work on assignments, and prepare for clinical practica, and try to get into this routine early in the semester.

There are many characteristics that make for a successful graduate student clinician. Knowing and developing these characteristics can help you get the most out of your first year of graduate study. To make sure that you make the grade, review Figure 7-2, which lists the characteristics of a successful graduate clinician.

Want to know if you have what it takes to be a clinician? See how well you match up with these attributes.

- *Dedication.* Your program of study is intensive and extensive.

- *Flexibility.* You need to have the ability to work with a variety of people in a variety of settings.

- *Teachability.* You must be willing to learn from others with different approaches and views.

- *Compassion.* This is a service-oriented profession. You need to demonstrate a caring attitude to those served.

- *Reliability.* Those served must be able to depend on your presence as well as your knowledge.

- *Persistence.* Keep working to find the best possible solution.

- *Curiosity.* Keep investigating causes and concerns.

- *Accountability.* Document your work and keep records.

- *Ethics.* You will address confidential issues on a daily basis. The clients, supervisors, and future employers must be able to rely on your ethical behavior.

- *Appropriate Behavior.* Develop the ability to interact with others in an appropriately professional manner. This includes your conversation and your appearance.

- *Academic Proficiency.* Trying to maintain a balance is difficult, but you must maintain adequate academic proficiency.

- *A sense of humor!*

**Figure 7-2** Characteristics of successful graduate clinicians *(Source: Delmar/ Cengage Learning.)*

## GET FAMILIAR WITH THE KNOWLEDGE AND SKILLS ACQUISITION FORM

American Speech–Language–Hearing Association's (ASHA) Council for Clinical Certification (CFCC) created the Knowledge and Skills Acquisition (KASA) form to document a student's acquisition of basic knowledge and skills as outlined in the standards for the Certificate of Clinical Competence (CCC). When applying for certification from the ASHA, students from Council on Academic Accreditation in Audiology and Speech–Language Pathology (CAA)-accredited programs must submit the KASA.

The KASA documentation certifies that the student has acquired the oral, written, and cognitive skills, along with the required coursework, needed to attain ASHA standards and earn clinical competency. The accredited graduate academic program will determine which courses are acceptable in providing the student with the prerequisite knowledge needed in biological and physical sciences, mathematics, and social/behavioral sciences.

Begin compiling your KASA documents after completing each semester. Maintaining the KASA folder after each semester will keep you organized and will lessen the chances of losing or misplacing reports and information that are required for certification documentation. Also, plan your academic coursework so that you can meet the observation requirements (375 hours for audiology majors and 400 hours for speech–language pathology majors). Take every opportunity that is available to get those hours completed.

More detailed information about the KASA is available on the ASHA Web site. Search for "KASA."

## GET ORGANIZED

Successfully getting through the first year of graduate coursework is directly related to getting and staying organized. Save all of your notes, handouts, and books because they will be valuable resources when you are an independent clinician and/or researcher. They will also help you when you prepare for The Praxis Series, which you have to pass to work in some states and to get ASHA certification. Set up a system for filing and storing these materials so you can easily access them if needed for another class, a clinical experience, or studying for The Praxis Series. Below are some easy-to-implement ideas to help you get organized and stay on track. For more information on organizational tools, see Appendix A.

### Purchase a Large Backpack, Rolling Computer Bag, a Tote Bag, and a Clothes Basket

As a graduate student, you will have many materials to carry with you. A normal-sized backpack may not be large enough. You will have many binders, textbooks, and therapy supplies, especially on days when you have more than one class and clients. You may want to consider an extra backpack with wheels, a rolling computer bag, a tote bag, and a clothes basket. The clothes basket may sound weird, but it is an excellent choice for carrying therapy supplies such as toys.

### Make a Timeline of Your Courses Now until Graduation

At the beginning of your program, you probably received a list of courses that you are required to take. In addition, there may be some electives you can choose. Often, universities only offer graduate courses once every academic year. Thus, planning early, in your first year, for courses you need, or want to take during the next few years, is a good idea. This approach will increase your chances of taking the elective courses that interest you the most. Create a timeline of what course you will be taking each semester until graduation. This timeline might change, but at least you will have an idea of what to expect each semester. Put this schedule in your binder with all other graduation-related papers.

If you went to an undergraduate institution that is different from your graduate institution, you should make an appointment with your graduate academic advisor to determine whether you are missing any courses required for the graduate program. If you are lucky, you may find that you do not have to take one or two courses because you completed them as an undergraduate.

## Organize Graduation-Related Papers in a Binder

At the beginning of your program, you may receive information about courses, teaching certification, ASHA certification, portfolio requirements, and thesis and/or dissertation requirements. You are likely to forget about the information once classes begin, but professors and classmates will occasionally mention the important information throughout your program. Having these papers in a special binder will make it easy for you to access the information when you have questions.

## Organize Your Class Binders for Future Use

In at least the first few years as a professional, you will periodically be referring to your class notes. It is important to realize this fact early on in your graduate life because you will probably want to organize your binders so they will be useful years later. As an undergraduate, you probably organized your binders under the categories "assignments," "notes," "readings," and so on. Although these categories helped you with staying organized as an undergraduate, they will probably not be very functional categories for referencing when you are a professional. For future use, organize your binders by specific categories related to a particular class, such as "child assessment," "child treatment," "adult screening," and "adult treatment." You may want to put subcategories, as well. For example, under "child assessment," you might add "standardized assessments" and "nonstandardized assessments." In addition to easy access to your class notes as a professional, binders also accommodate, for example, journal articles you have read and handouts you received from a conference.

## Make Daily and/or Weekly Lists of Tasks to Complete

Do not tell yourself you have too much to do and there is no time to make a list. Take 5 minutes to write down what you need to get done for a day or a week. Prioritize based on what is due first—complete a reading assignment, search for an article in the Internet, e-mail a professor, and so on—and depending on how you work, update the list as needed to stay on track. You may want to have a list of goals to be accomplished by the end of the day, week, month, semester, and year. Making a list and using it to stay organized is a good way to prevent those late-night worries from keeping you up. If you find yourself having a hard time falling asleep because you are worrying about all the things you need to accomplish, get up, make a list, and try to go back to sleep. You might be surprised by how making the list will ease your mind and how much easier sleep will come.

## Constantly Improve Your Time Management Skills

To avoid procrastination, students should improve their planning and efficiency skills. In graduate school, it is unlikely that a student will have a whole day to complete a single assignment. Instead of waiting until 6 hours before a lengthy assignment is due, students should work on assignments in smaller increments. They should take advantage of the 15 minutes between classes or the 20 minutes on the bus to get work done. (In 15 or 20 minutes, students can probably write a goal for a therapy report or learn a page of notes!)

## GET HELP IF YOU FEEL YOURSELF GETTING OVERWHELMED

When graduate school gets hectic, you may forget to take care of yourself. Get enough sleep, eat three healthy meals per day, work out at least a few times every week, and drink plenty of water to stay hydrated. Always carry a water bottle with you. Below are some additional suggestions for maintaining good self-care during your graduate program.

## Ask a Second-Year Graduate Student to Be Your Mentor

By making a concerted effort, at the beginning of each semester, to meet students in your classes, you will be building a wide network of support. Consider asking a second-year graduate student to be your mentor. Some graduate programs have a buddy system that is organized through the National Student Speech Language Hearing Association (NSSLHA) chapter. It is always easier to get through coursework when your peers are there for emotional and academic support. If there is no such program, consider starting one.

## Balance Your Coursework and Clinical Work

Designate time to read your textbooks, work on assignments, and prepare for clinical practica. Try to get into a routine early in the semester.

# Take Things One Hour at a Time

Say to yourself, "What do I want to concentrate on for the next hour?" Sometimes, you just need to take a deep breath and do what you can. Looking at all things to be accomplished during a week can get overwhelming. It may be beneficial to make a daily schedule of where you need to be and what you need to be doing each hour of the day. Focus on accomplishing things in smaller increments and you may feel more successful and less stressed.

# Complete Assignments Early

When you have a week where you do not have a lot of assignments due, get ahead for the following week. You will find that assignments are a lot easier to complete when you are not working under the stress of getting them done the day before—or sometimes the same day—they are due. Moreover, if you have questions on your assignments, you will have time to ask your professor. Using a lighter week to get ahead may keep an upcoming, potentially stressful, and hectic week more manageable.

# Be Open with Professors and Clinical Instructors When You Are Overwhelmed

If your coursework overwhelms you, be open with your professors. Let them know that you are trying hard. They may be expecting too much. They may change an aspect of the course if they realize that they have unrealistic expectations. If you are overwhelmed in part because of personal reasons outside of class, such as a death in the family or an illness, let your professors and clinical instructors know. They will probably be willing to provide you with extra support, or possibly let you take an incomplete grade if things are too overwhelming. Moreover, you may want to seek counseling services on campus to help you through difficult times.

# Take Advantage of the Educational Opportunities Offered

You will not have another time in your life when you will have faculty members readily available to teach you and answer your questions. Right now, if you have almost any question related to a client, you are just a phone call, e-mail, or appointment away from problem solving with a professor or clinical instructor. You may not have this same kind of support once you are in professional practice. Take advantage of all that your professors have to teach you!

Your department and university may offer a wide range of additional educational opportunities. Take advantage of continuing education courses to fine-tune your skills. Courses relating to computers, literature searches, and writing may be available through your university or a local community college. Graduate school is a wonderful time to gather information you will use every day when you are a clinician and/or researcher. Make the most of your time in graduate school.

## You Are Assessed Differently

Professors in graduate courses usually assess students' knowledge by giving essay examinations, case studies, group assignments, and writing assignments (or papers). Some papers may be 20 or 30 pages long, which is considerably longer than the types of papers written in undergraduate courses. Other papers may be limited to one page but must be written very concisely. Graduate classes are more likely to be interactive. Students are expected to ask questions and discuss assigned readings and material presented in class. Some courses may have a laboratory component. In many clinical practica, students are assessed by their interactions with their clients, preparation for sessions, and written reports. Unlike undergraduate courses, professors are less likely to use multiple-choice and short-answer tests. Be prepared to assess yourself, especially in the area of clinical practice. Many supervisors expect you to write a self-assessment before meeting with them to discuss your progress with your clients. Be prepared to objectively evaluate your clinical skills and point out areas of strength and areas for improvement.

## You Know More Than You Think You Know

Faculty members prefer students to express their ideas, as long as students have a reason for what they are saying. Sometimes, when a faculty member asks a student a challenging question, the student may respond, "I don't know because I have not taken a class on it yet." This type of response may cause frustration to the faculty member. Instead of focusing on what he or she does not yet know, a student should always try to answer the question based on what he or she does know. Furthermore, a student can follow-up an answer by stating how to find out more information or ask the faculty member a specific question that will help lead to a solution.

Much like the experiences students have in graduate school when approaching a new topic for the first time, clinicians and researchers will be faced with situations that are unfamiliar to them. However, those who pull from their previous knowledge and ask questions are more likely to effectively solve problems. Like students, faculty members reason and think their way through right and wrong possibilities. The sooner students realize that they need to consider several right answers, the more likely they will provide good care for their clients and solve research questions.

## There Can Be Many Right Answers to Problems

Most undergraduate courses use true-or-false and multiple-choice tests where there is only one correct answer to each question. Students are used to memorizing material, recognizing the "right" answers, and regurgitating what was taught. When these students enter graduate school, they soon discover that there is more than one "right" answer to a problem. In CSD, the *right* answer may vary based on: the case; the severity of a disorder; the client's personal, social, psychological, financial, religious, and cultural concerns; or increasingly, on what insurance or Medicare/Medicaid will cover. Likewise, within the field there are differing philosophies or theories of assessment, diagnosis, and treatment, and depending on the theoretical approach, the right answer to a problem may vary widely.

## Relax! Most Students Make It Through

Students should be comforted in knowing that it is extremely rare that someone does not make it through graduate school. These very few who do not make it through usually decide to take a different career path because the clinical experience was not what they thought it would be. These students usually did not have an undergraduate clinical practicum experience and, sometimes, choose to go into research psychology or another field without clinical practicum, but still related to health care. It is extremely rare for students to not make it through graduate school because of academic grades.

Students also need to realize that, in graduate school, decisions are rarely "life and death." Audiology and speech–language pathology are not like surgery. In general, clinical experiences are only extremely critical situations when working in intensive care or with patients who have dysphagia. Fortunately, when clinically related decisions need to be made that may result in life-or-death outcomes, students will be working with experienced supervisors. The supervisors will teach them how to sort through the difficult decisions they face.

## CONCLUSION

While in graduate school, continuously remind yourself why you are going through the obstacles and be grateful for the opportunities to take on the challenges. Remember that there is a light at the end of the tunnel. You will not be in graduate school forever. Before you know it, you will be a working professional helping people living with communication disorders and their families.

# Advice for the Final Year of Graduate School

## INTRODUCTION

After all your years of schooling and training, you are getting closer to your career as an audiologist, speech–language pathologist (SLP), or speech–language–hearing scientist. You will be busier than ever the year before graduation. It is around this time that you must find an externship, apply for The Praxis Series, apply for licensure, and apply for American Speech–Language–Hearing Association (ASHA) membership and certification. The key to getting through the final year of a graduate program is timing. This chapter provides you with a timeline to successfully move you toward your professional career. Figure 8-1 is a checklist for you to use to track your progress.

## TWELVE MONTHS BEFORE GRADUATION

### Consider a Clinical Fellowship or Externship Position

To become an ASHA-certified audiologist or SLP, you must complete a clinical fellowship (CF) or an externship after you graduate. Typically, speech–language pathology majors participate in a CF at the completion of the Master's program. Au.D. students end their fourth year of graduate study with an externship. For more detailed information about the CF and the externship, see Chapter 10.

The CF lays the foundation for the rest of your professional career. Take your time identifying a supervisor who is best able to provide you with support and encouragement through this period. More important, make sure that this individual is ASHA certified. It is during this time that you will be working and gaining the professional experience you need to receive your Certificate of Clinical Competence (CCC). Contact your department's clinic director/coordinator to find out who is responsible for arranging externship positions.

If you have to find externship positions on your own, there are several options to consider. If you have previous volunteer experience in a clinic, hospital, or school where audiology or speech–language pathology services are offered, these locations may be more receptive to taking you on as an extern. However, do not feel limited by your past experiences. You should seek out novel opportunities and consider contacting other places that you believe could offer beneficial experiences. If you are seeking ASHA certification, as

**Twelve Months Before Graduation**

☐ Consider what kind of Clinical Fellowship or externship position you would prefer

☐ If you are interested in research, inquire about research assistantships or hourly rate positions

☐ Join an ASHA Special Interest Division

☐ Consider doctoral study

**Nine Months Before Graduation**

☐ Start researching certification requirements

☐ Attend the ASHA convention, state convention, and other related conferences

☐ Participate in a poster session during the ASHA convention

**Six Months Before Graduation**

☐ Create a portfolio

**Three Months Before Graduation**

☐ Seek out and attend job interviews.

☐ Identify a clinical fellowship or externship position

☐ Prepare for the comprehensive examinations

☐ If you want to work in a school setting, make sure you know the requirements

☐ Start preparing for The Praxis Series

☐ Take The Praxis Series during your last semester of graduate study

**One to Three Months After Graduation**

☐ Start your new job!

☐ Apply for state certification and/or licensure after graduation

☐ Convert your membership from NSSLHA to ASHA

**Figure 8-1** Advice for final-year graduate students *(Source: Delmar/Cengage Learning.)*

you seek out externships, remember that your supervisor must hold ASHA's CCC. This point is so important it bears repeating twice.

## If You Are Interested in Research, Inquire About Research Assistantships or Hourly Rate Positions

If you are interested in learning more about research, identify a professor in your department who is conducting research that interests you. Because most schools have a limited number of assistantships, apply early if there is more than one deadline. Assistantship opportunities may vary throughout the year, as can the compensation for participation. For instance, a professor may look for a research assistant after receiving a grant during the middle of an academic year. Depending on the level of research needed, there can be a wide range of methods for compensating you for your time and effort. Keep your eyes and ears open throughout the year for assistantships. Be an advocate for yourself because professors are unlikely to seek you out to give you a job.

If assistantships are unavailable, ask about working for a professor at an hourly rate, such as a work-study position. Sometimes you can volunteer and earn academic credit. Working for a professor will allow the professor to get to know you. If and when the professor has an assistantship position available, he or she may be more likely to hire someone he or she knows. Furthermore, working with a professor, regardless of the position, will be a valuable learning experience.

There are assistantship programs beyond research assistant that can be valuable learning experiences and can help offset the cost of your education. These opportunities include teaching, clinical, and project assistantships. Ask your advisor for more information. You can also look on your department's Web site, and on department Web sites in related fields, such as psychology, communications, laryngeal physiology, and special education, for these opportunities.

## Join an ASHA Special Interest Division

As you are getting further into your graduate studies, you may have some specific interests that are guiding your studies. Start interacting with other individuals who share similar special interests. ASHA recognizes different divisions where members can affiliate with a network of professionals and students with similar interests. For more information on the Special Interest Divisions, see Chapter 26. Members of the National Student Speech Language Hearing Association (NSSLHA) are eligible to join a division for $10. Figure 8-2 is a list of 10 reasons why a student should join a Special Interest Division.

1. **Membership.** Membership is $10 a year for students. NSSLHA members can join any of the 16 divisions and receive all of the great benefits for only $10 a year.

2. **Listservs.** Interact with other division affiliated through members-only Listservs. Imagine having a direct line to experts representing the entire scope of practice.

3. **Members-Only Access.** When you join a division, you get members-only access to topic-specific materials online.

*(continues)*

**Figure 8-2** Ten reasons to join a Special Interest Division

4. **Web Forums.** Participate in Web forums, which attract leading researchers and practicing clinicians in the field. Forums may offer training on treatment techniques, discuss current issues, or even debate controversial topics.

5. **Perspectives Newsletter.** Each division publishes a newsletter, *Perspectives*, with division news, details on sponsored events, and articles on hot topics in the area of specialty.

6. **Preconference Workshops.** Divisions offer special pre-conference workshops on the day before the official start of the ASHA convention.

7. **Continuing Education Credit.** Many divisions have multiple opportunities to earn continuing education credit—not an issue for you as a student, but someday you will love your divisions for providing these options for continuing education.

8. **Additional Professional Topics or Areas.** Join professionals who participate in additional professional topics or areas that impact both speech–language and hearing. Special Interest Divisions: Division 11, Administration and Supervision; Division 12, Augmentative and Alternative Communication; Division 13, Swallowing and Swallowing Disorders (Dysphagia); Division 14, Communication Disorders and Sciences in Culturally and Linguistically Diverse (CLD) Populations; Division 15, Gerontology; Division 16, School-Based Issues.

9. **Audiology.** Join professionals spanning the scope of practice in audiology. Special Interest Divisions: Division 6, Hearing and Hearing Disorders: Research and Diagnostics; Division 7, Aural Rehabilitation and Its Instrumentation; Division 8, Hearing Conservation and Occupational Audiology; Division 9, Hearing and Hearing Disorders in Childhood.

10. **Speech–Language Pathology.** Join professionals who span the scope of practice in speech–language pathology. Special Interest Divisions: Division 1, Language Learning and Education; Division 2, Neurophysiology and Neurogenic Speech and Language Disorders; Division 3, Voice and Voice Disorders; Division 4, Fluency and Fluency Disorders; Division 5, Speech Science and Orofacial Disorders; Division 12, Augmentative and Alternative Communication; Division 13, Swallowing and Swallowing Disorders (Dysphagia).

**Figure 8-2** (*Continued*)

## Consider Doctoral Study

Why stop at the Master's level? Expand your employability and career options by obtaining a doctoral degree. Talk with your advisor about this degree and stop by the Graduate School Fair at the ASHA convention. Many doctoral programs offer significant scholarships and financial aid. Additionally, the job market looks extremely bright for individuals with a Ph.D. working in a university setting. If you are interested in research and/or teaching, you should consider a doctorate degree. You can read more information about doctoral study in Chapter 12. A list of ASHA-accredited doctoral programs is also available on the ASHA Web site. Search for "EdFind."

# NINE MONTHS BEFORE GRADUATION

## Start Researching Certification Requirements

Ask your academic advisor, mentor, or clinic instructor about state and ASHA certification requirements. Make a timeline of what you need to do during your graduate program to be eligible for certification when you graduate. Ensure that you keep your Knowledge and Skills Acquisition (KASA) summaries up to date and filled out correctly. Contact the Action Center at 800-498-2071 to evaluate your eligibility for the ASHA Conversion Discount. Now that you are moving toward being a professional, it is important to take responsibility for knowing these requirements and following whatever steps are needed to obtain them.

## Attend the ASHA Convention, State Convention, and Other Related Conferences

As a Master's student, attending these events will become even more important to your academic and professional development. More information about the benefits of attending the annual ASHA convention is available in Chapter 25.

## Participate in a Poster Session During the ASHA Convention

ASHA usually announces the Call for Papers (CFP) in January with an April deadline. Announcements will appear in *The ASHA Leader* and on the ASHA and NSSLHA Web sites. This is your opportunity to share your research with a captive audience. Take advantage of this platform and present what you have been working on at a poster session.

# SIX MONTHS BEFORE GRADUATION

## Create a Portfolio

Having a portfolio when attending interviews will make you stand apart from other applicants. Some employers, particularly schools, require a portfolio for an interview. Portfolios generally include written samples of your paperwork from different clinical settings, types of disorders you have worked with, examples of diagnostic and treatment tools used, state and national conferences you attended, national examinations you have passed, your résumé, and other relevant information. Some graduate programs require electronic portfolios, whereas other programs require paper portfolios. Ask your clinic director or an advisor about what specific information you should include.

## THREE MONTHS BEFORE GRADUATION
## Prepare for the Comprehensive Examinations

Some Master's programs require students to take comprehensive examinations (comps) before graduation. The comps are an examination that universities administer after the first year or during the last year of a Master's program to assess what students have learned. However, other programs use The Praxis Series instead of comps. Ask your advisor or the department chairperson whether your program has comprehensive examinations and when they are offered. Also, find out whether your program hosts meetings or reviews throughout the year to help students prepare for the comps. Attend these meetings and start studying early. Studying for both the comps and The Praxis Series around the same time is helpful because studying for one will prepare you for the other.

## Start Preparing for The Praxis Series

The Praxis Series is an examination designed by the Educational Testing Service (ETS) to assess the competency of audiologists and SLPs as they enter their fields. The examination is sometimes called *the ASHA Exam*, *the ASHA Boards*, or *NESPA* (an older term that is rarely used anymore). Audiology students must take the audiology version of the examination, and speech–language pathology students, the speech–language pathology version. The examinations cover material taught during undergraduate and graduate courses.

To become an ASHA-certified audiologist or SLP, students must score 600 or higher on the Praxis II. Most states require the same score for certification; however, some employers are only interested in scores higher than 600, such as 650 or 700. Students can repeat the examination, and Praxis does not average scores. ASHA does not offer a Praxis preparatory course; however, resources for preparing for the Praxis are available in the ASHA Web site. Start studying for the Praxis examination early in your final year of your Master's program.

If you are applying for ASHA certification, you are required to mail a copy of your Praxis report to ASHA. As part of a graduation requirement, your graduate program may require a report of your scores, as well. Ask your advisor if the department needs your scores.

## Take the Praxis

Many students choose to take this examination during their last semester of Master's study, although you can choose to take the examination earlier. Taking the examination earlier can relieve some anxiety because you know you will have a chance to take the examination again and prepare for the areas where you are weakest.

## If You Want to Work in a School Setting, Make Sure You Know the Requirements.

Most states require professionals to take a certain number of education and special education courses and have teaching experience. Some states require professionals to pass an examination related to special education. For instance, the Alabama State Department of Education has the Alabama Prospective Teacher Testing Program (APTTP): Basic Skills Assessment Test to assess readiness. The state of California requires the California Basic Educational Skills Test™ (CBEST®) to assess educators' basic reading, writing, and mathematics skills in the English language. The state of Pennsylvania uses the Praxis II Principles of Learning and Teaching Tests for grades K–6 and 7–12. Initial teacher certification with the West Virginia Department of Education requires the Pre-Professional Skills Tests (PPST) in reading, writing, and mathematics. For more details on individual state requirements, consult with your advisor, state board of education, and an audiologist or an SLP who currently works in schools.

## ONE TO THREE MONTHS AFTER GRADUATION

### Apply for State Certification and Licensure

Once you have successfully completed the Praxis examination, send your passing scores to the professional boards of your state for you to obtain state certification and licensure. Every state has different requirements for submitting the scores. Research your state's requirements for certification on the state association page of the ASHA Web site. Remember that it is your responsibility to know what type of certification or licensure is needed for the type of setting in which you will work. Do not assume that your employer will tell you what certification or licensure is required. You must independently and proactively fulfill all such requirements.

### Convert Your Membership from NSSLHA to ASHA

Students who maintain two consecutive years of NSSLHA membership qualify for the NSSLHA-to-ASHA Conversion Discount program. This discount provides a savings on the initial fees for membership and certification in ASHA. A significant number of students lose eligibility for the discount every year because they wait until the last minute to convert their membership. You do not have to wait until you complete your CF to apply to ASHA. You simply need to submit your application by August 31 of the year following graduation to apply at the reduced rate. If you are not sure whether you qualify for the Conversion Program Discount or when you need to convert your membership, contact the NSSLHA office at nsslha@asha.org before your Master's graduation date.

## Carefully Keep Track of Certification and Licensure Expiration Dates

As soon as you receive your temporary or permanent licenses and certification, write down when they expire, fees you have to pay to renew, and continuing education requirements. Never, ever see patients/clients if your temporary or permanant license expire! You could commit insurance fraud and face heavy penalty, including having your license revoked and not be able to practice. Apply for renewal well before the expiration date; sometimes, applications can take a month or two for a licensing agency to process. Don't hesitate to contact your licensing and certification agencies if you have questions.

## CONCLUSION

Depending on your course of study and your career goals (audiology versus speech–language pathology), your Master's program may be the final degree you will need before beginning to practice professionally, or it may be one more step toward acquiring your doctoral degree. This chapter provides excellent advice for keeping track of the many things to be accomplished as a second-year graduate student. The checklist in Figure 8-1 can be a useful tool for tracking your progress. If you have obtained your Master's degree, passed the Praxis, completed your CF, and applied for certification, you are ready to enter the job force, congratulations! You have made significant achievements during your communication sciences and disorders (CSD) studies and are about to embark on an incredible journey that will positively impact the quality of life for many people with communication disorders. If you are preparing to enter a doctoral program to continue your studies, congratulations to you as well! Your educational journey will continue to provide you with exciting new academic, research, and clinical experiences, which will help shape the future contributions you make to the field.

# CHAPTER 9

# Advice for Clinical Practicum

## INTRODUCTION

Beginning your clinical practicum is both an exciting and stressful time. Many students feel overwhelmed with thoughts of having to simultaneously complete assignments for classes and plan for clinical practicum. The practicum allows you to assimilate academic work into the real-world situations. You may be asked to evaluate new clients, develop and modify treatment plans, plan therapy sessions, or experiment with new therapy techniques. This chapter provides background information about the clinical practicum experience and advice to help you prepare for and succeed in your clinical work.

## BEGINNING YOUR CLINICAL WORK

Depending upon the university, students may begin their clinical experiences at either the undergraduate or the graduate level. The American Speech–Language–Hearing Association (ASHA) requires all students to complete a minimum of 400 hours of clinical work. Of these 400 hours, 25 hours are reserved for clinical observation and 375 hours must be direct contact with clients (with 325 of these hours to be completed at the graduate level). These hours must be completed under the direct supervision of a speech–language pathologist (SLP) who holds a Certificate of Clinical Competence. ASHA standards mandate that supervisors must periodically directly oversee at least 25% of the 400 hours over the course of the practicum.

Universities provide many options for clinical placements, including in hospitals, schools, rehabilitation facilities, nursing homes, early childhood development programs, and university clinics. You may be allowed to select the placement or the university department may assign these based on the availability of facilities or the areas in which you need to develop competency (see section on Documentation).

Training programs will have basic requirements that must be met before allowing students to begin their practicum experience. For example, you may be required to complete a criminal background check, have a physical or tuberculosis (TB) skin test, or provide a résumé. It is important that you do not wait until the last minute to meet these requirements. Delaying the completion of paperwork can delay the beginning of your clinical experience. Practicum facilities may also require specialized training or have other individual requirements, so be prepared to attend orientations and read all information sent to you from the practicum facility.

Punctuality is a crucial part of your clinical practicum. To allow for transportation delays and to prepare yourself for work, plan your arrival for at least 15–30 minutes before your assigned time. Delays can be unavoidable and absences do happen, but you should call your supervisor as soon as possible. Practicum sites are extending you the privilege to work and learn your profession; it is imperative (for both you and your program) that you meet scheduled obligations. Universities can lose practicum sites if a student does not take their obligations seriously.

Finally, you are a professional and it is important that you present yourself as one. Some facilities require dress codes (such as scrubs), and others may require business attire. It is advisable that you dress the way you want to be perceived by the client, family, caregivers, and your supervisor. Remember that first impressions can last forever.

## IT'S OKAY TO BE NERVOUS

Making a successful transition from traditional academic work to applied clinical practice is an essential part of the clinical practicum, but not necessarily an easy one. As a clinician, you may feel nervous, scared, or unsure of yourself and it is important to know that it is all right to have these thoughts. Much like starting a new job, you may have preconceived notions about what it will be like, but after the first day your experiences may have been completely different than first envisioned. You must realize that no one expects you to be perfect. The beauty of the profession is that you are afforded the opportunity to *practice*, and through this practice your nerves will calm and your confidence will grow.

## ESTABLISH A BOND WITH YOUR SUPERVISOR

Perhaps one of the most important parts of your clinical practicum experience is forming a bond with your supervisor. They are considered your teachers, but there should also be a reciprocal relationship. You may be able to inform them about new therapy practices or assessment instruments that you are learning about in class and they will be able to provide information from their years of experience. Be willing to learn from your supervisor and accept constructive criticism.

As you complete your externships outside of the university setting, remember that you may be placed in facilities that could consider you as a future employee. Show your supervisor that you are willing to work hard and go the extra mile. They may allow you to use them as a reference when you begin your search for employment.

## PREPARE FOR YOUR FIRST CLIENT

You will always remember your first client, especially if you see him in a clinical setting twice weekly for hour-long sessions. Whether you have a good experience or a not-so-good experience, there are a few things you can do to prepare for your first client.

## Plan Ahead

If paperwork is available, review your client's information. It is especially important to know their age and their diagnosis so you can plan appropriately. It is also helpful to develop a consistent way to record data (not just for writing session notes, but as a means for effectively monitoring treatment progress). Be sure to become thoroughly familiar with your institution's requirements for record keeping, including documentation of treatment effects and clinical hours. No matter how perfect you envision the first meeting to be, your clients may not be interested in the activities you had planned or they may not cooperate for the entirety of the initial evaluation. A college professor said, "Take lots of stuff," and this is to ensure that you will have a backup should things not go as you had anticipated. Figure 9-1 is a list of top-10 must-haves for audiologists.

1. **A Black Pen.** We have moved to electronic everything, but you are still going to have to write once and a while, and when you do, only black ink will do. And for the purists from the old school (right, round, red devotees), you will need red and blue.

2. **Audiograms.** The quandary is always two graphs or one. Regardless of your preference, chose one that is easy to read (by those other than the audiology staff); has a clear symbol key; and has places for patient identify information, speech testing scores, immittance results, and a signature. Develop your own, or take the easy way out and use a commercially available one, such as in the ASHA Practical Forms in Audiology product, available through ASHA product sales, 888-498-6699.

3. **Antibacterial Moisturizing Soap.** Everyone practices universal precautions, so after a few hundred patients your hands will look like lobster claws if you use only the standard antibacterial soap. Of course, there is always hand lotion to fix that, but why not kill two birds with one stone?

4. **Safety Goggles.** Ears may be our thing, but much that we do puts our eyes at risk. Good safety glasses can keep your eyes safe from airborne earmold modification materials, infectious material, and, of course, that proverbial spit in the eye. (Not all patients have Emily Post manners.) Gloves, gowns, and masks are also must-haves.

*(continues)*

**Figure 9-1** Top-10 must-haves for audiologists

5. **Distraction Devices.** Anyone who works with children must have a supply of simple toys that will grab a child's interest long enough for you to get that tympanogram done or that earmold impression taken. Toys that fit in the pocket of your lab coat are great. Bubbles are also an audience pleaser. Try hitting the local fast-food chains and ordering kids' meals. It's a cheap way to collect great toys—and an excuse to eat fast food!

6. **Resource Book.** Every audiologist should have a book with a list of local, state, and national resources. Compile a list of all the early intervention providers, support groups, advocacy organizations, funding sources, educational contacts, Web sites, counselors, and so on, in your area. You should also have at your fingertips the names and numbers of national organizations. The ASHA *Let's Talk Audiology* publications and the ASHA Web site (www.asha.org) are good places to start.

7. **Diagnostic Equipment.** Every audiologist needs a good audiometer, immittance bridge, sound booth, and otoscope just for the basics. But if you're going to do full-scale diagnostics, you'll have to add otoacoustic emission, auditory brainstem, and video nystagmography equipment. For hearing aid dispensing, you have to include real ear and hearing aid analyzer equipment, as well as a dedicated computer for fitting and tools for shell modifications. There are lots of fun toys in audiology!

8. **Commitment.** A commitment to human service is why we do what we do. There will be days when you doubt that commitment, but making a point to reaffirm your commitment will make you a better audiologist and more satisfied in your work.

9. **Computers.** You can't practice without computers that are dedicated to specific clinical applications, such as otoacoustic emissions (OAE), auditory brainstem response (ABR), videonystagmography (VNG), and hearing aid fitting. Plus, you'll need a computer for your patient database, scheduling, inventory, accounts payable and receivable, and so on. One has to wonder how we ever practiced audiology before we had the personal computer.

10. **Passion.** Be passionate about what you do! Your love of your work will be evident to your patients and colleagues, and it will come back to you 10-fold.

Reprinted with permission by the National Student Speech Language Hearing Association *NSSLHA Now!* April 2005.

**Figure 9-1** *(Continued)*

## Establish Rapport

One of the most crucial aspects of therapy with any client is the initial establishment of rapport. Be pleasant and polite. Let him know that you are available for questions because you are there to help. Making the client feel comfortable will make your job easier. It is also important to set behavioral limits that first day. It will be difficult to control nonproductive behavior if it is allowed to occur during the initial visit. To learn about your client before the first day of therapy, consult with your supervisor and read the previous therapy notes (if available).

## PARENTS, FAMILY MEMBERS, AND CAREGIVERS

When your client's parents, family members, or caregivers play an active role in therapy, your task is usually made easier and treatment is more effective. The important people in your client's life need to be kept well informed about the client's progress with therapy. Do not fear their questions about your therapy. View their questions as a representation of their good intentions and as an opportunity for you to practice your professional consultation. The more they know, the more they can help the client when you are not with the client and family members are doing therapy. You can provide resources to family members and take-home activities that reinforce therapy goals. It is important to be thankful when you get a parent who is considered "too involved" because it is much better than not being involved at all.

## BE FLEXIBLE

The world is not going to come to an end if your client does not do exactly what you want, and coming to this realization is a turning point in the clinical practicum experience. As a clinician, you must remember to be flexible. When something happens that is out of your control, becoming upset is not the answer. Perhaps it is most important to not interpret undesirable behavior as targeting you personally. The ability to adapt to unforeseen events can make a good clinician a better clinician.

## DON'T BE AFRAID TO ASK FOR HELP

Although you are now a clinician, you are still a student. You are continually learning about the profession and are not expected to know everything. However, you are expected to turn to others when you are asked questions and are unsure of the answers. It is better to ask for help than misinform family members. In some situations (like university clinics), parents and caregivers are paying discounted rates for students to provide services to loved ones with communication disorders. They are aware that you are still in training to become a future SLP or audiologist. Asking for help is part of the learning process.

Your supervisor is a great source of information, but it may also be possible to get ideas from fellow classmates and your professors. National Student Speech Language Hearing Association (NSSLHA) membership provides you access to all of the resources that ASHA provides for its members and is a tremendous resource for students. In addition, consider joining the Special Interest Divisions that are important to you. The Special Interest Divisions publish outstanding information for clinicians. For additional information, refer to Chapter 26.

# DOCUMENTATION

## Clock Hours

Most universities have developed their own system for tracking and storing information about the number of hours you have accumulated during your practicum experiences. However, systems fail and paperwork can be lost. For your peace of mind, you can develop your own system or keep duplicates of the training institution's records. You should keep copies of all paperwork related to your clinical hours and store them in the same place. Creating a simple spreadsheet on your computer and saving it in multiple locations (hard drive, flash drive, CD, etc.) is a quick and easy way to total and keep track of your clock hours. If there is ever a question about your time, you will have your own copies to which you can refer.

## Knowledge and Skills Acquisition Form

The Knowledge and Skills Acquisition (KASA) form is a record of competencies that you have demonstrated during your clinical practicum or through class projects. There are nine areas in which you must demonstrate competency in evaluation and intervention: articulation, receptive and expressive language, cognitive aspects, fluency, hearing, social aspects, voice and resonance, swallowing, and communication modalities.

Most universities require your professors or supervisors to submit in writing when you have met a certain competency (i.e., at the end of your practicum or upon the completion of a project for class). According to ASHA's 2005 Standards and Implementation Procedures for the Certificate of Clinical Competence:

> The applicant must adhere to the academic program's formative assessment process and must maintain records verifying on-going formative assessment. The applicant shall make these records available to the Council for Clinical Certification upon its request. Documentation of formative assessment may take a variety of forms, such as checklists of skills, records of progress in clinical skill development, portfolios, and statements of achievement of academic and practicum course objectives, among others.

This means that, as part of the certification process, ASHA requires all students to submit evidence that clinical training has been accomplished. This may take the form of the KASA or another written record that your training institution has developed. As your supervisors or professors confirm that you have met certain competencies, it may be helpful to fill in your own KASA form for your records.

As you approach the halfway point of your placement, it is advisable that you sit down with your supervisor and review your KASA (or alternative record) form. There may be times when you are having difficulty obtaining competencies in a specific area. When you sit down with your supervisor, you may be able to ask whether there will be any opportunities in which you can demonstrate competency in those areas. Supervisors can be very accommodating when helping students complete their KASA competencies. You can access the KASA online at ASHA's Web site. Search for KASA form.

## Résumé Information

Keep a record of any special treatment techniques or procedures that you learn. These may be valuable pieces of information to include in a résumé.

# RESOURCES

There is an abundance of therapy resources that you can use for planning sessions during your clinical externships. Also, many sources of materials for therapy are available, but for NSSLHA members, there is a wealth of information about current research, best practices, and theory available on the ASHA Web site.

## The ASHA Leader

ASHA publishes The ASHA Leader 16 times a year, and NSSLHA members have access to it. The ASHA Leader offers information on current research in the field as well as information about new therapy techniques and programs. It helps keep members updated on the most recent developments in speech–language pathology and audiology. The ASHA Leader also publishes a classified advertisement section for jobs, and there are many service providers who advertise here.

## NSSLHA Now! NSSLHA Now!

Is the newsletter of the NSSLHA. The newsletter is published three times per year: Winter (February), Spring (April), and Fall (November). The newsletter focuses on current issues affecting students and is written in a manner that is student friendly.

# Internet

Online resources continue to be of great assistance when planning therapy sessions. There are numerous Web sites (often developed by SLPs and audiologists) that offer worksheets, materials for activities, and interactive games. These resources are usually available free of charge or subscriptions can be purchased for a small fee. Take time to explore the Internet for materials that you may find useful for certain clients. Anyone can post on the Internet, so you will need to make certain that your materials are appropriate and that methods used are supported by the best evidence available.

## Class Texts and Presentations

During your college, you will probably be asked to give numerous presentations on various disorders, therapy techniques, new devices, and tests. Keep copies not only of your presentations but of those given by classmates. These are excellent resources to use when you have questions about, for example, what test to use with a client, what alternative and augmentative communication device may work, or what characteristics accompany a certain disorder. For easy reference, store this information in an organized manner.

Many students never sell their books from their speech–language pathology and audiology classes. Ask anyone in the profession if he or she has referred back to a classroom text and his or her answer will probably be yes. It is advisable that you keep your books, as well. They are excellent references to use when completing your placements. You may have questions about a certain client and be able to find the answer in an old textbook.

## *Advance* Magazine

*Advance for Speech–Language Pathologists & Audiologists* is a weekly publication that provides information about newly developed therapy techniques and research studies in the field. Subscribe to *Advance* online at http://speech-language-pathology-audiology.advanceweb.com/.

## CONCLUSION

As you learn more about clinical practice, you will become a better clinician. With each externship you complete, you will notice yourself feeling more comfortable with clients, family members, and caregivers. Though you may only see a client for a few months or even a few weeks, you will be making a difference. Your clinical placements should be both educational and enjoyable. The rewarding road to becoming an SLP or audiologist begins with your first clinical practicum experience.

# CHAPTER 10

# Advice for the Audiology Externship or Clinical Fellowship

## INTRODUCTION

If you want to practice professionally as an audiologist or a speech–language pathologist (SLP), you must complete a supervised clinical experience upon graduating from your program. If you are an audiology student, this period of supervised clinical work is referred to as an *audiology externship*. If you are a speech–pathology major, you will refer to this period as a *clinical fellowship* (CF).

For the most part, the experience is the same for both. However, there are a few slight variations, such as the number of hours required for certification and compensation. This experience is your first job out of graduate school, where you are still under the supervision of an American Speech–Language–Hearing Association (ASHA)-certified professional, as you were in the clinical practicum or rotations. However, you will be working and engaged in client treatment as if you are a professional.

This chapter provides an overview of the postgraduate clinical experience and what to expect during the clinical experience. Figure 10-1 lists some advice to help you prepare for your clinical experience.

**Make sure you have the necessary heath requirements, security clearances, and liability insurance**

Every site will have a different set of basic requirements that must be met before allowing students to begin their practicum experience. Find out through the interview process what your site will require. For example, you may be required to complete a criminal background check, have a physical or TB skin test, or provide a résumé. It is important that you do not wait until the last minute to meet these requirements. Delaying the completion of paperwork can delay the beginning of your clinical experience.

Some facilities require student clinicians to obtain liability insurance. Liability insurance is available to members of the NSSLHA at a discounted rate. For more information about this benefit, read Chapter 24.

*(continues)*

**Figure 10-1** Everything you need to know to prepare for your clinical experience *(Source: Delmar/Cengage Learning.)*

**Make sure you know the facility's policies and procedures**

Practicum facilities may also require specialized training or have other individual requirements. Be certain to attend orientations, and read all information sent to you from the practicum facility. Inquire about things such as dress code, call-in procedures for sick days, what to do in a patient emergency, and, of course, the Health Insurance Portability and Accountability Act (HIPAA) policies of the site.

**Clarify your work schedule with your supervisor**

Make sure that you understand when you are to report to work with the supervisor. Even though you are a student, the sites will expect you to show to work as any employee. Punctuality is a crucial part of your clinical practicum. To allow for transportation delays and to prepare yourself for work, plan your arrival for at least 15–30 min before your assigned time. Delays can be unavoidable and absences do happen, but you should call your supervisor as soon as possible. Practicum sites are extending you the privilege to work and learn your profession; it is imperative (for both you and your program) that you meet scheduled obligations. Universities can lose practicum sites if a student does not take their obligations seriously.

**Make sure that you understand what you will be doing**

Ask for a description of the caseload at the facility, especially if there has been no opportunity for a visit to the site for an interview and tour. It is not uncommon for students to be taken by surprise, thinking their placement was in a rehabilitation hospital only to find exclusively acute care patients on the caseload.

**Make sure you know what your supervisor expects**

Discuss the way supervision will be provided, including the frequency of direct observations, the plan for supervisor/supervisee conferencing, and the ways feedback will be provided by the supervisor. Do not assume it will be the same way as the university clinic supervisors do it. All supervisors must adhere to the minimum guidelines for supervision set forth by ASHA.

**Make sure you know what type of support you will have from your program**

What happens if you have difficulty during the externship? What types of intervention will be provided by the university?

**Make sure you know the paperwork you will be required to submit**

That means paperwork at the externship site—not the daily SOAP notes, Individual Education Plans (IEPs) or progress reports required by individual sites. Appendix C has information on clinical writing that may be useful.

**Figure 10-1** (*Continued*)

# THE AUDIOLOGY EXTERNSHIP

ASHA requires the completion of a 12-month full-time equivalent of supervised clinical practicum, called *audiology externship*, sufficient in depth and breadth to achieve the required knowledge and skills outcomes for students completing a doctorate of audiology (Au.D.) program. Students partaking in an externship refer to themselves as *externs*.

Students work with the clinical director or externship coordinator (the title varies among academic programs) to find externship placements.

Compensation during the externship is an ongoing debate. Paying or reimbursing externs for their services implies that externs are working and, thus, are employees, as opposed to being students under supervision. Some programs do not provide any monetary compensation and some do. Moreover, some extern sites require students to pay tuition fee while working on their externship because the extern is still considered a student. However, in this case, as students, externs will qualify for school loans to support them through the externship. In other cases, students should discuss with the clinical director or externship coordinator the financial aid options available to support the externship.

The American Academy of Audiology suggests the following timeline for selecting externship positions:

| | |
|---|---|
| Student/faculty search process | Students/faculty investigate program opportunities, requirements, deadlines; July through October |
| Application period open | Extern sites accept applications during this time period; September and October |
| Application submitted | Final date for sites accepting applications; October 31 |
| Applications files completed | Letters and transcripts to be on file; November 15 |
| Interviews | December and January |
| Offers made | Offers made by sites to students on February 1 |
| Accepted Round 1 | Offers accepted by students within 2 weeks |
| Follow-up offers completed | Process completed by March 31 |
| Externship begins | Between June 1 and July 1 |

# THE CLINICAL FELLOWSHIP

Speech–language pathology majors refer to their period of clinical work as a *clinical fellowship*. The term *CF* is also used as a noun to describe a person completing a CF because during this period you will refer to yourself as a *clinical fellow*. It is in the CF that you, for the first time, will truly practice most of what you have spent years learning.

ASHA requires all students to complete a minimum of 400 hours of clinical work for certification. Of these 400 hours, 25 are reserved for clinical observation and 375 hours must be direct contact with patients/clients (with 325 of these hours to be completed at the graduate level). These hours must be completed under the direct supervision of an SLP who holds a Certificate of Clinical Competence. ASHA standards mandate that supervisors must periodically directly oversee at least 25% of the 400 hours over the course of the practicum.

Some programs allow the graduate to select the placement, and others have staff, the clinical director, or CF coordinator to find placements based on the availability of facilities or the areas in which the students need to develop competency.

In most cases, the placement sites compensate CFs for the responsibilities performed.

## GUIDELINES FOR CHOOSING AN EXTERNSHIP OR CLINICAL FELLOWSHIP

You will flourish as a clinician if you are in a setting where you are comfortable and believe you are contributing to the good of your clients as well as the clinic. Figure 10-2 is a checklist for choosing a CF site.

### Consider Carefully What You Are Looking for in a Work Site

As you work in different settings during your internships and externships, consider what you do and do not like about each setting. Think about both what you can offer a site and what the site can offer you in terms of experiences. Talk to your supervisor about potential openings in the future. It is never too soon to consider your options.

☐ Consider carefully what you are looking for in a work site

☐ Start sending out résumés the semester before you graduate

☐ Talk to professors in your department

☐ Bring your portfolio with you to interviews

☐ Ask questions during the interview

☐ Figure out what qualities and work style you want most in a supervisor

☐ Consider the differences between settings

**Figure 10-2** Checklist for choosing a clinical fellowship *(Source: Delmar/Cengage Learning.)*

# Start Sending Out Résumés the Semester Before You Graduate

Send résumés to sites that have listed an opening, as well as sites that may not be hiring at this time. Many professional publications—such as *The ASHA Leader, NSSLHA Now!*—as well as many career-specific Web sites—such as ASHA's Career Center (http://careers.asha.org/search.cfm), Audiology Online (http://www.audiologyonline.com/careers/), and Advance for Speech–Language Pathologists and Audiologists (http://www.advanceforspanda.com)—advertise CF job openings. Realize that it may take 6 months to a year to find a job, depending on what cities you are searching. Be open to participating in a CF outside the area where you live or go to school. Sometimes the opportunities are in areas that will require you to relocate.

## Talk to Professors in Your Department

Professors in your department often have close friends and colleagues across the country who may know of CF openings. Sometimes, employers send job postings to university communication sciences and disorders (CSD) departments and your professors may have knowledge of these job openings or prospective employers. Your National Student Speech Language Hearing Association (NSSLHA) chapter may have a job binder that stores these postings. Use all the resources at hand to help secure a job once you graduate. The professors and resources in your department can be invaluable both now and down the road, if you maintain contact after graduation.

## Bring Your Portfolio with You to Interviews

It is especially important to bring any writing samples (e.g., research papers) to interviews. Your portfolio will give a potential employer a better idea of your capabilities. The portfolio will also help employers see that you are prepared for the interview.

## Ask Questions During the Interview

The interview is not only a time for the employer to determine whether you are a qualified candidate but also your opportunity to determine whether the position, employer, and setting are right for you. When you meet with a potential supervisor, feel free to ask questions in addition to answering questions. You are trying to find a good fit for both you and the employer. Do not be afraid to ask for what you want. When applying for a CF, consider asking your potential supervisor the following questions during the interview:

- What types of services are provided to clients?
- Are there best-practice rules or protocols in place?
- Approximately how much time will you commit to be accessible to me each day or week?

- Have you supervised a CF or extern before?
- Are you familiar with the requirements of a CF or externship?
- If you have not supervised a CF or extern before, have you worked with students at any level?
- Do clinicians have administrative time set aside, or are their schedules limited to clinic responsibilities?
- Are your audiologists and SLPs ASHA certified?
- Are you familiar with state licensure and certification requirements?
- Are you located solely at one site or do you manage many sites?
- Do you have rotating positions, or do you expect CFs or externs to work for this facility after the CF is complete? (Some sites have rotating positions. When that time is up, you move on to another position. Other sites will not want to invest the time to hire, train, and supervise a CF or extern without the probability that he or she will stay on after ASHA certification is attained.)
- What benefits are there? (Some professionals recommend that you ask this question once you are offered a job.)
- What is the average salary? (Asking for the salary range during the interview is different from negotiating the salary during the offer period. Wait to negotiate your salary until you have been offered the job.
- Is there a salary increase once certification is attained and/or a full license is attained? (Discuss, up front, what possibility there is for advancement. It is better to learn about these details early. Keep in mind that it can be difficult or impossible to negotiate salary increases once you are in a position; however, again, some professionals recommend asking this question after being offered a job.)

## Figure Out What Qualities and Work Style You Want Most in a Supervisor

Although you may not be working closely with your supervisor at all times, you do need to have a good relationship. Make sure that your supervisor is going to be someone who can further your professional interests. Consider whether the supervisor will meet your needs by asking about his or her work style, expectations of employees, and the characteristics he or she values most in an employee. The most important thing is to make sure your supervisor is ASHA certified. You are wasting your time in your CF position if your CF supervisor is not ASHA certified. Call the ASHA Action Center at 800-498-2071 to verify your supervisor's certification.

## Consider the Differences Between Settings

A larger clinic or hospital will generally offer a broader range of experiences and more interesting cases, but you may encounter more bureaucratic issues, or some facilities may be required to hire fully licensed clinicians. A smaller clinic or private practice may be easier to work with but might not offer the variety of experiences a new clinician would benefit from. Take your time to figure out what things matter most to you. This is the first step in your professional future; you do not get a chance to do it over. If you still cannot make up your mind, ask yourself the following questions after each interview:

- Was it clear what would be expected of me? Did this facility do a good job of helping me understand what my caseload would be and the level of responsibility I would have? If the answer is not obvious, it might be a sign that the facility is not organized or that the work environment is tenuous.

- Does this facility care about compensating its employees? What type of employee benefits will this position provide? How flexible is this work environment? Even if it cannot give me the money that I am asking for, is the facility willing to negotiate additional incentives to show that I am valued?

- Did my potential supervisor seem approachable and reasonable? (You will need a supervisor who can answer your questions and explain things clearly. Not everyone is an effective teacher or mentor in an applied setting like a clinic, hospital, or school. Consider how your potential supervisor responds to your questions.) Did he or she give me the information I needed? Does this person seem like someone who is good with conflict resolution? (You are likely to encounter at least some challenges.)

- Will I be working with multiple clinicians with diverse backgrounds? (It is invaluable to work with multiple clinicians and gain insight from their points of view.)

- Do I see myself working here after my CF is complete? If it is a rotating CF position, would I feel comfortable changing jobs at the end of my CF?

- What do I like the most about this CF position? What do I like the least?

- Would I work here for free? (Your reply to this question will really gauge if this is the right position for you. If you would seriously consider working in that setting free of charge, then imagine how great it will be to get a paycheck.)

## CONCLUSION

After many years of education and training, you are finally stepping into a professional role to provide services to individuals with communication disorders. This step forward is the start of what will likely be a long, successful, and enjoyable career. To get off to the right start in your CF, do your homework to determine what setting and employer is the right fit for you. Just as you did when you were applying to undergraduate and graduate programs, research your options and ask questions so that when the time comes to accept a position, you are positive that it is a job in which you will flourish.

# The Certificates of Clinical Competence

## INTRODUCTION

Once you have received your graduate degree, you will want to apply for certification in either audiology or speech–language pathology. Certification is a nationally recognized credential that is evidence that you are highly qualified to perform professional service. The American Speech–Language–Hearing Association's (ASHA) Council for Clinical Certification (CFCC) is responsible for the certification process. The CFCC defines standards that assure that the individual providing service has the "knowledge, skills, and expertise to provide high quality clinical services, and they actively engage in ongoing professional development to keep their certification current." This chapter covers the standards and maintenance requirements for audiologists and speech–language pathologists initially applying for certification.

Individuals seeking certification must complete a detailed application process. With so much going on around graduation time, students often delay the process by making common mistakes. Figure 11-1 provides some helpful tips to successfully complete the certification process.

Most people are unaware that membership and certification are two independent processes. A student may elect to apply for certification without being a member of ASHA. Equally, a student who is not engaged in the provision or supervision of clinical services may apply for membership without applying for certification. Applying for both membership and certification at the same time, however, ensures that you have all the resources that you need to function professionally and can also afford a savings in application fees. Students who maintain national membership in National Student Speech Language Hearing Association (NSSLHA) for 2 consecutive years at the time of graduation from their master's program are eligible for the ASHA Conversion Discount. The ASHA Conversion Discount provides students with a reduction in cost equivalent to the ASHA membership dues at the time of application. The discount is automatically applied when a student applies for membership and certification application.

## CERTIFICATION STANDARDS IN AUDIOLOGY

The certification standards in audiology require that applicants complete 75 semester hours of postbaccalaureate education, culminating in a doctoral or other recognized graduate degree, including academic coursework and a minimum of 12 months of full-time equivalent, supervised clinical practicum. The course of study must address the knowledge and skills pertinent to audiology.

### Completing the Application

- Read all instructions and sections of the application before completing. If the certification unit receives an application with any part of the application blank, it will turn down the application.

- Pages 1–3 must be submitted first to begin the application process. Page 3 must be an original, signed, and completed by the program director.

- The Clinical Fellowship Report and Rating form is used to document your clinical fellowship experience. This form may be submitted with your application or after your application has been submitted but cannot be submitted before receipt of your application.

### Payment

- Payment must accompany the submission of pages 1–3 of the application. ASHA provides discounts to graduates who have membership in the national student association, NSSLHA. Contact the Action Center at actioncenter@asha.org to determine your eligibility for discounts on the initial dues and fees for ASHA membership and certification.

- Certification is granted once all standards have been met and full payment has been received.

### Submitting the Transcript

- Submit an original graduate transcript with the conferral date listed. Transcripts requested before the graduation date may not have the conferral date listed. It is best to wait until you have graduated to request your transcripts. Your school may send your transcripts to the certification unit or you may include them with your application.

### The Praxis Series Examination

- Students taking the Praxis examination must list ASHA as a recipient of your examination score each time you take the exam. ASHA will only accept examination scores submitted through ETS. ASHA's ETS code is R5031.

- The test must be taken until it is successfully passed.

- Scores achieved more than 5 years before submission of the certification application are not acceptable for certification purposes.

*(continues)*

**Figure 11-1** Tips for completing the application for the certificate of clinical competence in audiology or speech–language pathology *(Source: Delmar/Cengage Learning.)*

**The Clinical Fellowship**

- Before deciding on a clinical fellowship (CF) mentor it is recommended that you check with the Action Center to verify that your mentor is currently certified by ASHA in the area in which you are seeking certification.

- The CF will not count toward certification if your mentor is not currently certified.

- You may apply for ASHA membership and certification before completing the CF. As a matter of fact it's preferred. As a *member-in-process*, you have access to all ASHA membership benefits.

- Double-check that you have filled out the Clinical Fellowship Report and Rating form completely and that you and your mentor have signed the form in all sections requiring your signatures.

- Clinical Fellowship Report and Rating forms signed before the end of the CF experience may result in the clinical fellow being credited with less time than actually completed. Do not sign the form before ending your CF.

- Be sure to indicate the **hours worked per week** for Section 5 on the Clinical Fellowship Report and Rating form, **not the percentage of time for the week**. Partial weeks do not count.

- Submit a separate report and rating form each time you change sites, mentors, or hours per week. If you wait until your CF is complete, mentors may have moved and you may not be able to locate them for the corrections.

- If you change mentors, we recommend that you have the Clinical Fellowship Report and Rating form completed on the last day of your assignment with the first mentor. Submit the form to the certification unit and then start your new position with your new mentor and a new Clinical Fellowship Report and Rating form.

**Additional Information**

- Before submitting any paperwork to the National Office, **make a copy for your records**. We retain the originals only until certification is granted. Once certification is granted, copies of the application, the Clinical Fellowship Report and Rating form, and examination scores are destroyed.

*(continues)*

**Figure 11-1** (*Continued*)

- If you apply more than 3 years after graduation, you will need to submit both a graduate and an undergraduate transcript (else you will not be considered a pass-through).

- If your examination scores were achieved or clinical fellowship was completed more than 5 years before your application for certification is submitted, you will be required to repeat these as part of the certification process.

- Your application will be evaluated under the standards that are in effect when you apply and not on those in effect when you received your degree. For example, individuals who graduated before the 2005 SLP standards taking effect had until December 31, 2005, to apply under the previous 1993 standards. Applications received from January 1, 2006, forward were evaluated under the 2005 certification standards even if applicants had received their degrees between 1993 and 2006. In many instances, this procedure meant that the applicant was required to take additional coursework or complete additional clinical practicum hours to meet the 2005 standards.

- Once certification has been granted, you will be required to participate in the Certification Maintenance Program, which requires annual payment of fees and completion of 30 hours of professional development every 3 years. Your first certification maintenance interval will begin on January 1 of the year following the awarding of your initial certification; that is, if you become certified on July 15, 2009, your first certification maintenance interval is January 1, 2010, through December 31, 2012.

**Figure 11-1** (*Continued*)

The standards require that applicants have a foundation of prerequisite knowledge and skills, including:

- Skills in oral and written or other forms of communication
- Skills and knowledge of life sciences, physical sciences, behavioral sciences, and mathematics, demonstrated through transcript credit for a course in each of the four areas

Additionally, applicants for certification in audiology must have acquired knowledge and developed skills in four areas: foundations of practice, prevention and identification, evaluation, and treatment. Moreover, these standards require assessment of the student's acquisition of the specified knowledge and skills by the graduate academic program. Clinical practicum must include direct observation, guidance, and feedback by the supervisor to permit the student to monitor, evaluate, and improve performance and to develop clinical competence. Supervisors of practicum that will be used for ASHA certification must hold current ASHA certification in audiology. There is no postgraduate clinical experience required for ASHA certification in audiology. Applicants for certification are required to successfully complete the Praxis Series examination in audiology and to have their passing examination score submitted to the ASHA National Office by the Educational Testing Service (ETS).

The second phase of the audiology standards will become effective January 1, 2012. As of that date, all applicants for certification in audiology will be required to have a doctoral degree. For ASHA certification purposes, the degree can be a Ph.D., an Ed.D., a Sc.D., or the Au.D.

More information on the audiology standards is located on the ASHA Web site. Search for "audiology certification standards" on the site.

## CERTIFICATION STANDARDS IN SPEECH–LANGUAGE PATHOLOGY

The current speech–language pathology certification standards became effective January 1, 2005. These standards mandate 75 semester hours of coursework overall, including at least 36 semester hours at the graduate level. The program of study must address the knowledge and skills pertinent to speech–language pathology. Further, the standards require that the applicant have transcript credit in each of the following areas:

- Biological science
- Physical science
- Mathematics
- Social/behavioral sciences

Speech–language pathology applicants must demonstrate knowledge of basic human communication and swallowing processes, including their biological, neurological, acoustic, psychological, developmental, and linguistic and cultural bases. The applicants also must demonstrate knowledge of the nature of speech, language, hearing, and communication disorders and differences, and swallowing disorders, including the etiologies, characteristics, anatomical/physiological, acoustic, psychological, developmental, and linguistic and cultural correlates in nine areas. Moreover, applicants must demonstrate knowledge of standards of ethical conduct, processes used in research and integrating research principles into evidence-based clinical practice, contemporary professional issues, in addition to knowledge of certification, specialty recognition, licensure, and other relevant professional credentials. As in audiology, applicants for certification in speech will be required to possess skills in oral and written or other forms of communication.

With regard to clinical practicum, applicants are required to complete a minimum of 400 clock hours of supervised experience in speech–language pathology. Of those, 25 hours must be spent in clinical observation and 375 hours in direct client contact. Of the 375 hours of client contact, 325 must be completed while engaged in graduate study, and individuals holding current ASHA certification in speech–language pathology must supervise all hours used for ASHA certification.

After completing the academic coursework and supervised clinical practicum, applicants must successfully complete a Speech–Language Pathology Clinical Fellowship (SLPCF). This experience must consist of the equivalent of 36 weeks of full-time clinical experience with a mentoring speech–language pathologist who holds current certification in speech–language pathology. And finally, applicants for certification under the standards will be required to pass the Praxis examination in speech–language pathology.

Detailed information on the speech–language pathology standards is on the ASHA Web site. Search for "SLP certification standards" on the site.

## CERTIFICATION MAINTENANCE

Individuals holding ASHA certification are required to maintain that certification through annual payment of dues/fees and through participation in continuing professional development activities. The renewal period is 3 years, and the renewal mandates the accumulation of 30 hours of continuing professional development during each renewal period. This requirement applies to all certificate holders, regardless of the date they originally became certified.

*Professional development* is defined as any activity that relates to the science and contemporary practice of audiology, speech–language pathology, and speech–language–hearing sciences, and results in the acquisition of new knowledge and skills or the enhancement of current knowledge and skills. Certification maintenance requirements for both audiology and speech as well as FAQs are on the ASHA Web site. Search the Web site for certification maintenance.

## CONCLUSION

Although the standards for certification are detailed, the benefits of certification are many:

- Certification is the public's assurance that an individual has met rigorous, peer-developed, and reviewed standards endorsed by a national professional body.
- Employers welcome and respect certification by a national body.
- Certification limits liability claims.
- Certification is a fundamental standard among major health professions in the United States.
- Certification is important for internal professional recognition, external verification, and accountability.

For over 75 years, ASHA has been the guardian of the professions of audiology; speech–language pathology; and speech, language, and hearing sciences. Take the time to learn about the ASHA certification program and you will see that it is the symbol of quality.

# CHAPTER 12

# Doctoral Degrees and Selecting a Doctoral Program

## INTRODUCTION

In Chapter 2, we provided an overview of the job outlook and salaries for audiologists and speech–language pathologists (SLPs). As the data suggest, a positive job outlook exists for individuals with a doctorate. The profession is facing a critical shortage of SLPs and audiologists with entry-level degrees to assume faculty positions in communication sciences. There is a serious need for a next generation of individuals with these credentials. Developing more highly trained professionals who are passionate about research and clinical disorders ensures the longevity of the discipline.

Students pursuing doctoral degrees in the communication sciences are typically oriented in one of two directions: research or clinical. The coursework in a research doctoral program is directed toward a career as a teacher, researcher, or scholar, whereas individuals pursuing clinically oriented degrees focus on providing direct services and treatment to clients. Choosing one degree type over another depends on an individual's future career goals.

This chapter provides an overview of the coursework from each type and tips on how to apply to a doctoral program. Additional resources on doctoral degrees in communication sciences and disorders (CSD) are available on the Web site of the American Speech–Language–Hearing Association (ASHA). Search for "pursuing a Ph.D." The site has extensive resources on considering and preparing for a Ph.D. Moreover, this site is an excellent resource on everything from presenting your doctoral research to identifying funding for research projects.

## RESEARCH DEGREES

The doctorate of philosophy, or Ph.D., is a post–entry-level research degree awarded in recognition of published academic research and supported by a thesis or dissertation. The coursework covers a variety of research experiences and qualifying examinations. Some CSD programs combine the Ph.D. with a clinical course of study. The doctorate of speech–language pathology (SLPD) merges academic research with extensive clinical components.

The Ph.D. is not the only type of research degree that is recognized for certification in the discipline. Programs have the flexibility to structure the coursework of their advanced degrees to match the mission of the department. Below are other degree designators that you may find in a research program:

- **Sc.D., Doctorate of Science.** The Sc.D. is a research doctorate that includes the same academic coursework as the Au.D. coursework. Candidates complete a clinical practicum experience and a clinical residency (or externship). Sc.D. candidates are required to take interdisciplinary courses related to scientific and professional writing, statistics, research methods, biomedical ethics, and issues in health care.

- **Ed.D., Doctorate of Education.** The Ed.D. degree is often used in programs that are administratively housed in a school of education. The coursework in this program prepares the student for academic, administrative, clinical, or research positions in education and/or related fields. The Ed.D. is recognized by the National Science Foundation as equivalent to the Ph.D., because the requirements for both are similar. Some programs offer an Ed.D. with coursework concentrating on CSD; however, there are other Ed.D. tracks that focus on CSD-related areas. The Ed.D. tracks related to CSD include (a) *developmental studies*, which specialize in language and cognitive development; (b) *disability studies*, which address the needs of people who have language, speech, hearing, and/or cognitive impairments; and (c) *evaluation/assessment studies*, which focus on differential diagnosis instrumentation and procedures. These are but a few of the specialties addressed within this degree. As with the Ph.D., students are required to conduct research and develop a dissertation.

## CLINICAL DEGREES

The doctorate of audiology, or Au.D., is an entry-level degree designed for individuals who intend to specialize in the clinical practice of audiology. The Au.D. is required for audiology certification by ASHA. The first three years of a program generally consist of coursework and practicum, and the last year of study is spent completing an externship.

The Au.D. is not the only clinical degree recognized in this profession. As in the research degrees, some CSD programs offer an SLPD. The SLPD is the common degree designator for the post–entry-level clinical doctoral degree in speech–language pathology. The SLPD coursework combines academic research with extensive clinical research.

## SELECTING A DOCTORAL PROGRAM

Regardless of the degree designator assigned by the academic program, the ultimate goal is the degree. To become a certified audiologist or SLP, you must receive a degree from an accredited program. ASHA has developed an online, on-demand, academic program search engine—EDFIND—to help you easily identify accredited graduate CSD programs. A search of the ASHA Web site will yield access to EDFIND.

Prospective doctoral students have another outlet for researching graduate programs. The Graduate School Fair (GSF)—cohosted by National Student Speech Language Hearing Association (NSSLHA) during the annual ASHA convention—is a place to meet face to face with faculty from over 80 clinical and research doctorate programs in one venue for the cost of the registration fee. Members of the student association receive significant discounts to attend the ASHA convention, among other benefits. More information about the discounts and the GSF is available on the NSSLHA Web site.

The decision to get a doctorate is a big commitment because pursuing a doctoral degree means more time completing coursework and more educational expenses. Therefore, selecting a program that is the best match for you professionally and academically is important, which makes the selection process intensive. The department wants an individual who can advance the program's academic credibility. To be successful, you need a program that shares your passion for research and clinical advancements. The department will want to review your academic portfolio and interview you to learn more about your intention and focus. Similarly, you will want to know how the program is going to support your academic interests. The following are some of the questions that prospective programs may ask:

- Are you interested in basic or clinical research?
- What academic, clinical, and research experiences do you have, if any?
- What topics do you want to investigate?
- Do you want to be a professor?
- What teaching experiences have you had, if any?

Your decision-making process has to be just as intense. Before making your decision, visit the campus and view the facilities that will be shaping your academic interests. Get the viewpoint of students already enrolled in the doctoral program or who have recently graduated from the program. This is a great opportunity to verify the information you have gathered, to obtain advice on what your application materials should look like (especially your statement of interest), to get a feeling of what being a student in this program is about, and to identify any challenges students have had and how to address them. When interviewing with the department, make sure that your decision will be assisted by knowing the following:

- What type of research is the program engaged in?
- How many doctoral students are currently in the program?
- What kind of financial assistance exists for doctoral students? Tuition reimbursement? Research/teaching assistantships? Grants? Scholarships? Conference travel? How stable are the available funding sources? Will there be any obligations attached to funding during my time in the program or after graduation?
- How long does it take most students with my educational background (e.g. bachelor's and/or master's) to graduate?

- Will I get a list of current and/or recent alumni to contact about your program?

- Will I be required to study full-time or will I be able to continue working while I study?

- Would I be able to have mentors from outside your department or your academic institution on my committee?

- If I did not complete a master's thesis, will I need to complete an equivalent as a doctoral student?

- Will there be opportunities or obligations to teach undergraduate courses?

- What kind of coursework will I take? Are there required courses? Can I take courses outside the department?

- Does the institution require any culminating projects or comprehensive examinations?

A culminating project may be a small research study or literature review. Most comprehensive examinations either are lengthy tests that take 4–8 hours to complete or may come in the form of a written examination that requires the student to answer several in-depth questions over several weeks after all coursework and predissertation research projects (if any) have been completed.

## THE PH.D. SHORTAGE

Hearing, speech, and language scientists form the foundation of audiology and speech–language pathology by increasing or improving the knowledge base of the discipline. The profession needs these researchers to:

- Further investigate the neurophysiological, neurobiological, and physical processes that underlie normal communication

- Find new tools and techniques to prevent, identify, assess, and rehabilitate hearing, speech, and language impairments.

- Examine the role of cultural diversity in human communication, clinical perspectives, and approaches

- Explore causality and progression issues related to genetics, heredity, environmental, and social factors

- Work with clinicians to design and implement both medical and behavioral treatment protocols for hearing, balance, speech, language, and swallowing disorders (American Speech-Language-Hearing Association, n.d.).

There is a severe shortage of research scientists in the United States. Less than 1% of ASHA members and affiliates listed research as their primary function of employment (American Speech-Language-Hearing Association, n.d.). Currently, many faculty members are reaching retirement age, and there are not enough new Ph.D. candidates to fill their positions. In a survey of Ph.D. programs, the mean age of Ph.D. faculty was 49 years. Across the United States, there were 333 unfilled spots in Ph.D. programs ("PhD Program Survey Results

2002," n.d.). The employment prospects for individuals with doctoral degrees interested in performing research and teaching at a university are excellent.

# THE FINANCIAL COMMITMENT OF A DOCTORAL DEGREE

For many, obtaining a doctoral degree is a big financial commitment. On the basis of a recent survey, however, 86% of CSD doctoral students received funding. There was a large range of funding granted to these students. The average levels were $14,730 for extramurally funded Ph.D. trainees or fellows; $13,550 for extramurally funded research assistants; $13,320 for university-funded research assistants; and $11,360 for university-funded teaching assistants. Sixty-four percent of Ph.D. students received a full tuition waiver, and 19% received a partial waiver ("PhD Program Survey Results 2002," n.d.). The wide availability of funding, along with the excellent job market for individuals with a doctorate, is excellent news to individuals considering a doctorate in audiology or speech–language pathology.

More detailed statistics of the salary levels for audiologists and SLPs are in Chapter 2.

## CONCLUSION

By the time you apply to a doctoral program, you probably have gone through the academic application process many times and may feel quite comfortable with it. Some of the procedures and requirements are similar to what you may have done before. However, because the level of commitment to a doctoral program is more intense, the information schools are looking for from potential candidates may also be more extensive. As always, locate a program that fits well with your interests and goals. To have the greatest possible chance of gaining admission and funding to your chosen program, determine its specific requirements for admission early and make sure you provide everything needed, as asked for, on or before schedule.

## REFERENCES

American Speech-Language-Hearing Association. (n.d.). *Fact sheet: Speech, language, & hearing science.* Retrieved July 28, 2009, from http://www.asha.org/careers/professions/slh.htm.

American Speech-Language-Hearing Association. (n.d.). *PhD program survey results 2002: Executive summary.* Retrieved July 28, 2009, from http://www.asha.org/students/academic/doctoral/phd_survey_sum.htm.

American Speech-Language-Hearing Association. (1994). *Selecting a doctoral research education program in communication sciences and disorders.* Rockville, MD: Author.

National Student Speech Language Hearing Association. (November 2005). Top 10 considerations for selecting a graduate program. *NSSLHA Now!,* p. 6.

# CHAPTER 13

# Information About Postdoctorates

## INTRODUCTION

A postdoctorate period (also referred to as *postdoc*) is a unique opportunity for a recent Ph.D. graduate to focus on a specific area of research and to strengthen research skills. Postdocs generally span a period of 1 or 2 years and are typically funded by grant money obtained by a faculty member. This faculty member may serve as the recent Ph.D. graduate mentor during the postdoc period. Participating in postdoc research affords the Ph.D. graduate an opportunity to spend time exclusively on research without teaching, supervising, or committee responsibilities that typically accompany a faculty member position.

## PURSUING A POSTDOCTORATE

The following are some reasons to pursue a postdoc experience:

- To gain more research experience before applying for a tenure-track faculty position.
- To increase the number of articles accepted by peer-review publications.
- To expand skills and techniques in the research area.
- To learn how to effectively organize and manage a research project/facility.
- To gain knowledge/experience in a different research area.
- To increase funding opportunities from governmental agencies, such as the National Institutes of Health (NIH).

## FINDING A POSTDOCTORATE POSITION

What is great about a postdoc is that the Ph.D. graduate can sometimes create his or her own position under the supervision of a faculty researcher or clinician. The following is some advice on how to find a postdoc position:

- Check university Web sites for listings of postdoc positions in the communication sciences and disorders (CSD) department.
- Consider earning a postdoc in a related field, such as psychology or cognitive neuroscience.

- Search the Web sites of organizations such as the American Speech–Language–Hearing Association (ASHA) and the NIH.

- Network when going to conventions and conferences. Look for people in your area of interest who have completed a postdoc or are in charge of a program with a postdoc position available.

- Ask your advisor from your Ph.D. program for assistance in searching for a postdoc position.

## CONCLUSION

If you are on track to receive your doctorate and are interested in research, one of the most valuable experiences you can have is working as a postdoc. While focusing exclusively on research, you can develop the foundation for presentations and publications and can hone your research skills. Once you take a position as a professor at a college or a university, your attention will almost always be divided among teaching and advising responsibilities, committee work and department responsibilities, and research. For many, the postdoc experience is a singular opportunity to devote one's time and attention solely to research.

# PART 3

# Advice for Special Populations

# CHAPTER 14

# Advice for Parents of Students Applying to Graduate Communication Sciences and Disorders Programs

## INTRODUCTION

As parents, we wish for our children to be happy and fulfilled with their career choices and life's circumstances. Raising them to be productive and independent adults has been both a joy and a challenge, and guiding and supporting them through many decisions along the way has been gratifying. Now, as your child enters adulthood, she is also ready to consider her next steps in pursuing a career in communication sciences and disorders (CSD), applying to a master's degree or a doctoral degree program. This chapter will address some of the issues pertaining to parents' roles in this sometimes daunting process.

Admission to graduate programs in CSD is very competitive, and not all who seek admission will be successful. Assisting your child in searching for appropriate programs, navigating the application process, and handling the outcome (acceptance or denial) will be the topics addressed.

Information about the professions in speech–language pathology and audiology is available on the American Speech–Language–Hearing Association (ASHA) Web site. The "Students" link will give the reader an opportunity to explore the professions and information about career paths within CSD. To provide maximum support to students through their application processes, parents are encouraged to review this information.

The clinical entry-level degree required to become a certified speech–language pathologist is a master's degree, whereas the entry-level degree to become a certified audiologist is currently a doctoral degree. Programs in CSD that award MA, MS, M.Ed., MHS, among others, lead to certification in speech–language pathology. Moreover, many SLPs choose to pursue doctoral degrees as well, including the Ph.D., Ed.D., and SLPD (a clinical doctoral degree), although these degrees are currently not a requirement for certification in the field. The Au.D. is the designator for the clinical doctoral degree in audiology. A student may also choose to purse a Ph.D., Sc.D., Ed.D., or DA (doctorate of arts), which will also enable the graduate to become a certified audiologist if the academic and clinical requirements for certification have been satisfied.

# INVESTIGATING A COMMUNICATION SCIENCES AND DISORDERS PROGRAM

It is during the second half of the junior year in college that your child may need assistance in formulating a time line to explore various possibilities for graduate school, if he hopes to enter graduate school directly after earning the bachelor's degree. However, not all students take this formerly traditional route. Many now elect to take a break after four hard years of undergraduate study, to travel, to consider their options, or to just reenergize themselves. This chapter will revisit this second option later on.

Most graduate degree programs have application deadlines in the fall or early winter season. Therefore, juniors in college need to make use of the spring and summer preceding those deadlines to investigate programs and decide which ones they would like to apply to. Some programs have *rolling admissions*. In rolling admissions, there are no set deadlines for receiving applications; rather, the program reviews applications on an ongoing basis and considers students for admission for the next opening. Many programs start new groups of students only for the fall semester of each year, but others start students in the spring (January) semester and some even in the summer semester, as well.

EDFIND—ASHA's online, on-demand, academic program search engine—is an excellent place to start. EDFIND gives an overview of all CSD programs by the area of study, location, financial support, distance education options, among others.

Of note, in EDFIND, the option "Include only CAA accredited programs" is checked by default, which ensures that only those programs that have been reviewed and approved by the Council on Academic Accreditation in Audiology and Speech–Language Pathology (CAA) are listed. Graduation from a CAA-accredited program is one of the criteria that must be met in order for your daughter or son to eventually be granted Certificate of Clinical Competence (CCC) by the ASHA.

Details about programs listed on this site include a Web site address for each program and, usually, a contact person's name and e-mail address or telephone number. If you are helping your child with the legwork, go to the program's Web site and gather information for your child to read. The prospective applicant, not the parent, must e-mail and/or call the contact person with questions. This is the first contact the university will have with your child, and first impressions should be of an independent, self-confident thinker. Make sure that your child has read thoroughly the information on the Web site before contacting the program with questions. Asking questions that are already clearly explained on the site gives the impression that the student is not reading carefully and is not a good use of time for the busy program administrator or advisor who will answer the telephone call. Most Web sites do contain explicit information about application procedures (and even the application to be downloaded), an outline of the curriculum and course descriptions, and tuition and fees—print them out, bookmark them, and store them in folders in your desk drawer for future reference; you could also store this information on your computer's hard drive.

Even before beginning to search, check if your child needs help setting priorities for selecting programs. Factors such as distance from home, tuition and fees, and admission criteria are the obvious ones. Other considerations that may not be so obvious are the following:

- Are classes offered during the daytime, or during the evening, or both?
- Can the student hold a job while also going to school for the master's degree?
- Can the student take the program on a part-time basis, or does this program require full-time enrollment?
- What is the length of time required to complete the program? (Master's degree programs in speech–language pathology will not take as long to complete as doctoral programs for audiology certification.)
- Are students enrolled as a "cohort," or does each student progress through the program at his own pace?
- Is there a campus-based clinic as part of this program, or is all practicum done in off-campus locations?
- Does the program expect the student to attend classes and participate in clinical practice year round? (Most graduate programs do!)
- What is the size of the faculty and their various areas of expertise?
- If the student is interested in pursing a particular area of research, is this program able to accommodate and support this interest?
- What is the program's passing rate on The Praxis Series examination?
- What preparation does the program have in place to help students prepare for taking the Praxis?
- What types of extracurricular activities do students at this program typically become involved with? (Does the program have an active National Student Speech Language Hearing Association [NSSLHA] chapter?)

Do keep in mind that these questions are not value judgments. For example, programs that do have university-based clinics are not "better" than those who do not! These are just questions to help you and your child gain a better understanding of the overall structure of the program.

Once your child has narrowed down the search and has settled on a list of schools that she meets the established admission criteria, ask if she plans to visit the program. Especially if the program is far away, ask if he wants you to come with to help with the driving and to look at the town. For the sake of economics, you may want to wait to schedule a visit until your child has received a letter of acceptance and has made a decision about the enrollment. Or, your child may want to visit programs before an admission decision has been made, in order to participate in a face-to-face interview with a member of the faculty or admissions committee. NSSLHA hosts a Graduate School Fair at every ASHA convention. For the cost of the convention registration, your child will have access to over 80 academic programs in one location.

# APPLYING TO A MASTER'S SPEECH–LANGUAGE PATHOLOGY OR DOCTORAL AUDIOLOGY PROGRAM

Most program Web sites allow you to download applications directly, or even apply electronically. If your child is having difficulty getting started on applications, help your child organize the applications by deadline. Making a chart or spreadsheet is a good idea, with the name of the program, deadline for application, and columns for each piece of the application:

- The application itself, with the applicant's identifying information
- Official transcripts, from everyplace students have taken college level work
- Essays
- Letters of recommendation—many programs require that the student use their forms for this purpose
- Graduate Record Examination (GRE) scores—required by many programs, but not all
- Other items, such as a letter of intent, curriculum vitae, certificates, awards, which may be included with an application packet
- Address to which these items must be mailed
  - Sometimes it is to the program itself, but other times it is to a university's admissions office
- Interview

Once you have helped your child organize the application materials, you may discuss with him what other support he would like from this point on. Remember, as an adult, the student should take responsibility for the major portion of this application process, not the parent. However, there is nothing wrong with the parent helping the child to stay on track with deadlines and create a schedule for completing and submitting application materials. Additionally, you could proofread (not write!) essays and other materials before your child finalizes them for submission.

## PREPARE YOUR GRADUATE FOR THE INTERVIEW

Many programs require applicants to participate in a personal interview. Our professions require excellent interpersonal and communication skills, and the interview is one important way for the programs to evaluate those qualities of their applicants. Most programs do not interview all applicants but instead short-list candidates based on the programs' grade point average (GPA) and GRE requirements for the next round of admission interviews. Some programs require interviews to be done in person, and in those situations, you can help your child decide whether or not to travel to the school. If the student no longer favors the program because he was accepted to another program that meets his criteria, it would not be a good use of his time or the school's time to go for the interview. There are programs, however, that allow interviews over the telephone if students live at a significant distance from the school.

For face-to-face interviews, parents will certainly accompany their child to the meeting place but should not expect to participate in the interview. If a tour of the facility is offered, parents should inquire whether they can join in the tour (and most of the time they can). After the tour has been completed, the parent may either wait in the lobby or leave the facility and arrange for a later pickup time once the interview is completed.

Professional dress is recommended for the interview. Jeans, collarless T-shirts, flip-flops, and bare midriffs are not appropriate attire for interviews, even though students may have dressed this way throughout their college experience. Parents should advise their children about appropriate interview attire. It is not necessary to go to a great expense to purchase new clothing for the interview—just make sure the attire is neat and professional looking.

Whether the interview is in person or on the telephone, as parents, you can help your children prepare for the interview in several ways:

- Instruct your child to read the program's Web site and other information about the program before the interview. It makes a very good impression on the interviewer when the prospective student is knowledgeable about the program.

- Instruct your child to prepare questions beforehand, to ask the interviewer. During the interview, when the applicant says she has "no questions," it gives the impression that she is not very interested in the program and that she has not done any preliminary research into the program.

- Help your child prepare a mental list of important points that she wants to make sure the interviewer knows about her. For example, if your daughter was the president of the undergraduate NSSLHA chapter at her college, that is important for the interviewer to know. The prepared list will ensure that she brings that point up sometime during the interview. These points should also be included in a résumé that the applicant should prepare and submit with the application.

- Your child may want to rehearse the interview with you. Prepare a set of mock, generic questions, such as "What made you interested in pursing this career?" so that your child gets used to answering in complete, coherent sentences. Sometimes this mock interview helps calm some nerves, but other times it makes for increased nerves, so read your child carefully before embarking on this type of rehearsal with them.

# LIVING THROUGH THE ADMISSION DECISION

Programs vary in the way they notify applicants of admissions decisions. A growing number of programs send e-mail or have applicants log onto a Web site to get the decision. Others still send letters through the U.S. mail, with this important information. Usually, most programs will not give this information over the telephone.

As tempting as it is to be the "first to know," you owe it to your child to allow him to be the one to receive the news. He will certainly share it with you, and you will be there for him to either celebrate or console him in the case of a "denial."

When applicants are denied admission to the program they had listed as their first choice, it is disappointing to both them and you as their parents. This is where you play a major supportive role. Being visibly disappointed for a prolonged period of time will exacerbate your child's unhappiness. Not only will children take your reactions as their model for their own behavior, they will be doubly disheartened because they may misinterpret your empathy as actual disappointment with them.

Acknowledging your child's feelings is necessary and appropriate. Be empathetic but also be positive in reaffirming your child's worth and presenting a plan for further action, by saying something like, "I know how disappointed you are that you did not get admitted to … university's master's or doctoral degree program. Your qualifications are outstanding, and this is a very competitive process. Let's consider some of the other programs you applied to now, and look forward to hearing from them soon."

If your child is lucky enough to be admitted to more than one program, this would be a good time to narrow down the choices by personally visiting some of the schools. Your child should call or e-mail to ask for an appointment to visit the school and the specific program. This time, it is appropriate for the parent to accompany the child to the appointment. This meeting is different from an interview for admission—this time, it is a fact-finding visit, after the child has been granted admission to the program. Parents may have questions that will affect the decision about matriculation, including financial questions and living arrangements for the student. However, parents should take a backseat during the meeting and allow the student to direct the discussion most of the time. It is, after all, their future!

## GIVE YOUR GRADUATE A BREAK

Taking time off between college and applying to graduate school is a popular trend now, and for some parents, it is difficult to understand or accept. However, many students need this time to "find themselves," and this does not mean that your child will give up the idea of pursuing graduate education. The Peace Corps, Teach for America, and Studying abroad are excellent options for graduates to purse before deciding to continue their formal education. Others choose to seek unrelated employment for a year or two in order to save up money to assist with graduate school tuition and expenses. Many students who elect this route do apply and matriculate into graduate school with renewed energy and enthusiasm for the career path they have chosen! The maturation and self-confidence they gain from the break outweigh the year or two they have delayed in pursuing their life's passion.

## CONCLUSION

Parents can be of great help to their child during this stressful time, but they should be mindful of not taking over what their child should be doing: making her or his contacts and decisions. These young people are smart and savvy, and need your encouragement and confidence in their abilities.

As your child approaches graduation from college, she will be close to, or already have turned, 21. Legally, as an adult, it is your child who should communicate with the university programs. You may certainly contact schools to ask questions, but information specific to your child's application status, grades, and so on can only be shared with the student who is of legal adult age.

# CHAPTER 15

# Advice for Adults Returning to College to Pursue a Communication Sciences and Disorders Degree

## INTRODUCTION

Returning to school as a single parent was a huge decision. After a few years of working in a local public school and as mother to two young boys I decided to make a change in my life and return to school pursuing a master's degree in speech pathology. This academic journey has been extremely rewarding and challenging at the same time. I now have a different view on the importance of education and enjoy the impact academics and raising children have had in my life.

—*Sherri Webster, master's student, speech–language pathology, Western Washington University, Bellingham, WA*

Often the decision to return to school after years on your own—whether working a career or raising children—can be a difficult choice. Luckily you will find yourself in good company. It is not uncommon to find career-changers accepted in communication sciences programs. One of the traits that make for a good clinician is having a breadth of experiences. Career-changers bring diversity of perspective to the program.

—*Christine Neumayer, master's student, speech–language pathology, Lehman College, Bronx, NY*

This chapter offers some tips that may help adults returning to college after taking time away from school get the most out of their communication sciences and disorders (CSD) education. Figure 15-1 is a checklist of things to do to help ensure success.

## KNOW YOUR PROGRAM'S GENERAL REQUIREMENTS AND DEVELOP A PLAN FOR FULFILLING THEM

About half of a bachelor's degree consists of general university requirements (GURs) (also known as *general requirements, university studies program,* among other names). Primarily, GURs consist of courses in mathematics, biological and

- [ ] Know your program's general requirements and develop a plan for fulfilling them
- [ ] Get familiar with the knowledge and skills acquisition form
- [ ] Know your state's licensing requirements
- [ ] Balance your family life
- [ ] Be who you are
- [ ] Take advantage of learning resources early in your academic career
- [ ] Develop a study system that works for you
- [ ] Seek out resources for adults returning to college
- [ ] Take things one day at a time

**Figure 15-1** Checklist for adults returning to college *(Source: Delmar/Cengage Learning.)*

physical sciences, English, writing, behavioral and social sciences, and, possibly, foreign languages. Although many students complete these general course requirements at their 4-year college as part of their bachelor's degree studies, some adults returning to college may choose to complete GURs as part of an associate's degree from a community college or through an online degree program. Students sometimes choose to complete GURs at a community college because classes are less expensive and the community college environment can be smaller, geographically closer, or less intimidating than at a college or university.

If you are attending GUR classes at a community college, make sure that those credits can be transferred to the college you plan to attend. Some colleges or universities may not recognize credits taken at a community college as fulfilling specific university requirements. (This nonrecognition is due to many factors, so it is important to contact the CSD program's registrar's office to know how this nonrecognition affects you.)

## GET FAMILIAR WITH THE KNOWLEDGE AND SKILLS ACQUISITION FORM

The American Speech–Language–Hearing Association's (ASHA) Council for Clinical Certification (CFCC) created the Knowledge and Skills Acquisition (KASA) form to document a student's acquisition of basic knowledge and skills as outlined in the standards for the Certificate of Clinical Competence (CCC). Familiarity with KASA is important because students from Council on Academic Accreditation in Audiology and Speech–Language Pathology (CAA)-accredited programs must submit the KASA when applying for certification from the ASHA. This document certifies that the student has acquired the oral, written, and cognitive skills, along with the required coursework, needed to reach ASHA standards and earn clinical competency.

According to ASHA, the accredited graduate academic program will determine which courses are acceptable in providing the student with the prerequisite knowledge needed in biological and physical sciences, mathematics, and social/behavioral sciences. If your GURs do not transfer to your bachelor's degree or meet your university's KASA criteria, you will need to retake the courses, which will cost more time and money.

Moreover, ASHA requires students completing a degree in the communication sciences field to complete 25 hours of clinical observation. Complete these hours while you are completing your GURs or undergraduate coursework, when there are more opportunities for clinical observation. With these hours completed, you will relieve a bit of excess stress you will find your classmates faced with during the master's program.

You should begin compiling your KASA documents after completing each semester. Maintaining the KASA folder after each semester will keep you organized and will lessen the chances of losing or misplacing reports and information that are required for documentation.

More detailed information about the KASA is available on the ASHA Web site. Search for "KASA."

## KNOW YOUR STATE'S LICENSING REQUIREMENTS

In addition to GURs and KASA requirements, specific states have requirements that need to be fulfilled to practice as an audiologist or a speech–language pathologist. Most state requirements are easily fulfilled through coursework taken toward the GURs or bachelor's degree. Some states require you to complete a certification test. Being aware of what requirements are needed to practice in your state can aid in planning your academic pathways.

## BALANCE YOUR FAMILY LIFE

Deciding to return back to school is a huge decision. This decision is even harder when there are children or a family to care for. Finding a balance between maintaining your own academic career and the well-being a part of your family can be tricky. This balance only occurs when a routine is established. You must be realistic in your expectations of a routine and realize your own limits. Do not be afraid to ask for help and voice your concerns. Acknowledging your fears and concerns about balancing a family and school will aid in establishing the routine that is needed. Other tips for creating balance include the following:

- **Plan your childcare accordingly.** Look into childcare at your campus. Many schools have childcare and afterschool programs at a reasonable rate for students with children. Do this early! There may be a waiting list for entrance.
- **When you are with your children or family, focus only on them.** This activity may seem like common sense, but you will find yourself faced with a large amount of work; thinking about assignments that need to be completed and tending to your family's needs simultaneously

will be too overwhelming. Your children deserve your undivided attention. Make your time with them only about their needs. For the time being, put your coursework in the back of your mind and have fun with your family!

- **Make time for you and your spouse on a regular basis.** During your time together, have a date either in your house or out of it. Stay in and make a fancy dinner together. You could also ask your spouse to pick up a nice meal from a restaurant while you study and then enjoy the meal at home. As a study break, go for a walk for 20-30 minutes together, or if you have children, go to the park together and talk while your children play. On occasion, see if you can get away for a weekend with your spouse and go somewhere you have never been. This difficult time juggling your home life and school life will end. Within a few short years, you will have a regular 9AM–5PM job and will see your spouse more often; just don't fall into the trap of becoming strangers until that day comes!

- **Seek help from a high-school student.** It may be helpful to find a high school student to help your children complete their homework. During this time, prepare dinner, do housework, or read summaries in your textbooks for an upcoming class. This extra time, even if it is only an hour, will be a stress reliever for you and make for smoother transitions with your children at home.

- **Know your limits.** If you, because of sheer exhaustion, are unable to complete schoolwork assignments or readings after the children go to bed, make it a point to sleep and get up extra early and complete them before the day starts. Acknowledging your limits allows you to manage your time wisely and provide you with a feeling of accomplishment when your assignments are completed.

## BE WHO YOU ARE

You may feel self-conscious when most students are younger than you are. Remind yourself that you can learn something from everyone, regardless of age. Having more life experience puts you in the position to mentor younger students. Share your personal and professional experiences; you may have a lot to say that adds to the class discussion.

## TAKE ADVANTAGE OF LEARNING RESOURCES EARLY IN YOUR ACADEMIC CAREER

Recognize that it is not a weakness to admit that you need help learning how to learn. If you have been out of school for several years, you may have forgotten the study skills that many of your fellow students take for granted. Most colleges have learning centers to help you sharpen your study, reading, and comprehension skills. Many colleges have tutors for hire. All professors should have office hours where you can receive one-on-one help. Even the "A" students seek out tutors and learning centers to enhance their skills. Make use of all the resources available at your academic institution to help you learn and achieve your goals. Seek out additional resources as well, such as the ASHA and NSSLHA, websites which can help you become a successful student and professional.

## DEVELOP A STUDY SYSTEM THAT WORKS FOR YOU

You are responsible for your own study habits, and it takes time to develop systems that work best for you. Consider trying some of the following study skills:

- If you complete reading assignments before lectures, you will feel more prepared, and you can contribute better to class discussions.
- Use a highlighter to pinpoint the key ideas in your reading assignments or write key ideas in the margins. If you are pressed for time, skim over the chapter before class and try to understand the main ideas.
- If your textbook has chapter objectives and summaries, pay close attention to this material, as they will help identify the key points from the reading.
- Make a study guide or flash cards for material discussed in class within 24 hours of the lecture. By putting things into your own words, you also take ownership of the material, which helps you retain it in your long-term memory.
- Experiment with different ways of taking and reviewing notes. Record your class lectures; then as you are preparing dinner or driving in the car, listen to the lecture over again. You will be surprised as to how much you may have missed while trying to take notes in class and how much more sense the material makes.
- After you have reviewed material, consider forming a small study group and talk about what was learned. A study group allows for the opportunity to learn from each other. A classmate may have a different view on a topic or an approach you may not have considered. Being able to discuss material with another classmate shows that you really own this material; you will find yourself extremely confident participating in discussions and taking your examinations.

As you learn more about yourself and what kind of learner you are, you will be able to create an effective, personal study system.

## SEEK OUT RESOURCES FOR ADULTS RETURNING TO COLLEGE

As an adult returning to college, you are not alone! There are resources available to help with a wide range of concerns that are particular to this special population of students. Back to College (www.back2college.com) is a Web site with a comprehensive list of resources, scholarships, and services for adults returning to college. Register for their bimonthly electronic newsletter to access additional resources not listed on their Web site.

## TAKE THINGS ONE DAY AT A TIME

At times, your CSD program may seem more challenging than anticipated. You may have a demanding job or family that needs you in addition to your coursework and observation. You may feel it is too much. However, most things in life that seem overwhelming are, in fact, achievable if you believe in yourself, stay focused, take things one day at a time, and remember to ask for help when it is needed.

## CONCLUSION

For adults returning to college, the experience can be frightening, exhilarating, and challenging all at once. Some of the younger students sharing your classes may have the luxury of free time or freedom from other obligations, such as jobs or families, but may lack the experience you bring to discussions or the determination you have to achieve your academic and professional goals. Reminding yourself that the reason you chose to return to school is to better yourself with a rewarding and fulfilling career. Individuals happy with themselves and the choices they make will be a better provider within their family life and CSD career path. To achieve success in your CSD studies, make use of the resources discussed in this chapter and seek out other returning adult students to create a support system for yourself.

# CHAPTER 16

# Advice for Students from Culturally and Linguistically Diverse Backgrounds

## INTRODUCTION

The profession of communication sciences and disorders (CSD) is in dire need of individuals to assist in the delivery of services to the increasing numbers of individuals from multicultural backgrounds with speech, language, or hearing problems. Individuals with bilingual skills are especially needed as audiologists. Moreover, speech–language pathologists are mandated in many instances to provide services in the native language(s) of their clients. Currently, only about 2% of American Speech–Language–Hearing Association (ASHA) members are bilingual (see Figure 16-1).

Students interested in pursuing courses of study in these professions may want to increase their bilingual skills through participation in immersion programs and taking advanced courses in a foreign language. Students with multicultural or bilingual experiences and familiarity in working with racial/ethnic minority populations will be more marketable as these populations increase in numbers and become a larger proportion of the client population. This chapter discusses what you and other students from culturally and linguistically diverse backgrounds can do to stay competitive. Figure 16-2 offers a checklist to track your progress.

## ASK QUESTIONS ABOUT THE DIVERSITY OF THE FACULTY AND STUDENTS WHEN APPLYING TO AN ACADEMIC PROGRAM

When investigating potential CSD programs, ask about diversity in both the faculty and the student population. It is all right to ask the number of faculty that represents culturally and linguistically diverse backgrounds. It is also all right to know what resources the program provides to students from culturally and linguistically diverse backgrounds. Do not be afraid to ask these questions because you need to feel comfortable with the students you are going to network with and the professors who are going to train you for your career. Make sure that your graduate or undergraduate program is going to be a place that is supportive.

| | CCC in Speech | CCC in Audiology | Dual CCC | Certified Subtotal | In Process | Not Certified | Total |
|---|---|---|---|---|---|---|---|
| **Ethnicity** | | | | | | | |
| Hispanic or Latino | 2,155 | 149 | 13 | **2,317** | 37 | 15 | **2,369** |
| Not Hispanic or Latino | 64,776 | 7,049 | 596 | **72,421** | 596 | 312 | **73,329** |
| Not specified | 47,041 | 5,575 | 637 | **53,253** | 1,381 | 288 | **54,922** |
| **Total** | **113,972** | **12,773** | **1,246** | **127,991** | **2,014** | **615** | **130,620** |
| **Race** | | | | | | | |
| American Indian/ Alaska Native (only) | 192 | 20 | 1 | **213** | 2 | 1 | **216** |
| Asian (only) | 1,043 | 188 | 17 | **1,248** | 19 | 29 | **1,296** |
| Black or African American (only) | 1,798 | 139 | 10 | **1,947** | 28 | 7 | **1,982** |
| Native Hawaiian/ Other Pacific Islander (only) | 82 | 8 | 0 | **90** | 3 | 0 | **93** |
| White (only) | 62,256 | 6,663 | 559 | **69,478** | 591 | 274 | **70,343** |
| Multiracial | 1,621 | 205 | 19 | **1,845** | 8 | 14 | **1,867** |
| Not specified | 46,980 | 5,550 | 640 | **53,170** | 1,363 | 290 | **54,823** |
| **Total** | **113,972** | **12,773** | **1,246** | **127,991** | **2,014** | **615** | **130,620** |

**Figure 16-1** ASHA constituent counts by ethnicity, race, and certification status, January 1 through December 31, 2007 *(Source: ASHA Summary Membership and Affiliation Counts, 2007 year end.)*

☐ Ask questions about the diversity of the faculty and students when applying to an academic program

☐ If English is not your first language, enroll in English as a second language class

☐ Do not be afraid to admit you are having a problem keeping up with the coursework

☐ Gain experience working with culturally and linguistically diverse populations

☐ Participate in poster sessions and submit articles for publishing

☐ Search for financial aid opportunities for the culturally diverse

☐ Use resources available from ASHA's office of multicultural affairs

☐ Connect with a multicultural constituent group, caucus, or other organization

**Figure 16-2** Checklist for students from culturally and linguistically diverse backgrounds *(Source: Delmar/Cengage Learning.)*

# IF ENGLISH IS NOT YOUR FIRST LANGUAGE, ENROLL IN ENGLISH AS A SECOND LANGUAGE CLASS

Most campuses and major cities have courses for English-language learners (ELLs). These courses often include reading and writing skills enrichment. Let your professors know that English is not your first language and that you are continually working to improve your writing and speaking skills. Ask your faculty and peers for feedback on your progress in writing and speaking. Remember that proficiency in Standard English, although generally not a specific requirement, will be an advantage in widening your range of clinical options after graduation. If you are an ELL or speak a dialect other than Standard English as your native dialect, take every opportunity to improve these skills.

# DO NOT BE AFRAID TO ADMIT YOU ARE HAVING A PROBLEM KEEPING UP WITH THE COURSEWORK

If you are struggling with your coursework, especially if you are an ELL, seek help. If needed, ask for additional time to complete assignments appropriately and accurately. Let your professor know that you are continually working to improve your English reading and writing skills. Ask your professor questions if you are unclear about the requirements for an assignment. If allowed, work with a classmate on assignments so that you can teach each other and complete assignments efficiently. Also, most schools offer free tutoring services. Find out about these options at your school.

# GAIN EXPERIENCE WORKING WITH CULTURALLY AND LINGUISTICALLY DIVERSE POPULATIONS

Once enrolled in your course of study, take advantage of every opportunity to gain insight into and expertise in the provision of services to multicultural populations to increase your potential contributions to the professions. During your breaks from school, consider volunteering in clinics in developing countries. If this option is not feasible, consider getting a summer job as a tutor for children whose native language is not English or work in a hospital where there is a diverse population. If you have a choice about what public school, hospital, or clinic you can go to for a clinical experience, try to choose the place that has more diverse populations. When you work with clients who do not speak a language you know fluently or near fluently, you will need to know the procedure for finding a translator for your sessions. Talk with your clinical supervisor as needed for assistance.

# PARTICIPATE IN POSTER SESSIONS AND SUBMIT ARTICLES FOR PUBLISHING

As you consider topics for assignments and projects, think about researching topics that are related to culturally and linguistically diverse populations. Use your research to add to the proliferation of research, assessment and therapeutic techniques, and philosophies relative to communication disorders within bilingual and minority populations. Share your work by participating in poster sessions at student conferences sponsored by your CSD department or in CSD departments of other schools, at state speech–language–hearing conventions, or during the ASHA or National Black Association for Speech–Language and Hearing (NBASLH) conventions. NBASLH is open to all ethnic and racial groups. Also consider submitting papers to professional journals for publication.

## SEARCH FOR FINANCIAL AID OPPORTUNITIES FOR THE CULTURALLY DIVERSE

Your goal should be finding aid that will provide you with funding to meet all of your expenses. Many academic programs are participating in campus-wide initiatives for increasing diversity, and others simply have a desire to train professionals from diverse backgrounds. As a result, there may be scholarships, grants, or other forms of financial aid available specifically for ethnically and culturally diverse students. Ask your undergraduate or graduate program director or talk with the financial aid office at your school about these funding opportunities. Figure 16-3 provides a list of national organizations offering financial aid for diverse student populations.

---

- **The National Black Graduate Student Association, Inc. (http://www. nbgsa.org).** The National Black Graduate Student Association, Inc. (NBGSA), works to address African American students' needs and concerns in college and graduate school.

- **The Hispanic Scholarship Fund (http://www.hsf.net).** The Hispanic Scholarship Fund (HSF) is the nation's leading organization supporting Hispanic higher education and is committed to providing opportunities for students. For more information on the HSF, visit their Web site.

- **National Council of La Raza (http://www.nclr.org).** The National Council of La Raza (NCLR) works to increase opportunities and decrease discrimination and poverty among Hispanic Americans. NCLR has a Hispanic Scholarship Fund Institute for students who are Hispanic.

- **United Negro College Fund (http://www.uncf.org).** The United Negro College Fund (UNCF) is the nation's largest, oldest, and most successful minority higher education assistance organization.

---

**Figure 16-3** National organizations offering financial aid for diverse student populations *(Source: Delmar/Cengage Learning.)*

# USE RESOURCES AVAILABLE FROM ASHA'S OFFICE OF MULTICULTURAL AFFAIRS

ASHA has a unit of the National Office devoted to diversity and multicultural issues. ASHA's Office of Multicultural Affairs (OMA) provides technical assistance to its members and students in search of information and resources related to communication disorders in multicultural populations, as well as service delivery to those individuals. A detailed list of resources available from the OMA can be found on the ASHA Web site.

# CONNECT WITH A MULTICULTURAL CONSTITUENT GROUP, CAUCUS, OR OTHER ORGANIZATION

There are many groups and organizations that provide support services to students. Figure 16-4 provides a list and brief description of each ASHA caucus and other organizations related to culturally and linguistically diverse populations.

The following is a list and brief description of each caucus or other organization related to culturally and linguistically diverse (CLD) populations. Links to the ASHA-recognized Multicultural Constituency Groups are available on the ASHA Web site.

- **ASHA Special Interest Division 14.** The ASHA Special Interest Division 14 on Communication Disorders and Sciences in Culturally and Linguistically Diverse (CLD) Populations provides continuing education materials, networking opportunities, and mentoring opportunities for students.

- **Asian Indian Caucus.** The Asian Indian Caucus (AIC) promotes collaboration of knowledge and research about individuals who are Asian Indian.

- **Asian Pacific Islander Caucus.** The Asian Pacific Islander Caucus works to increase the number of students who are Asian Pacific Islander (API) and discusses issues related to professionals, clients, and students who are API. This caucus works to increase other professions' awareness of working with API clients who are receiving audiology, speech, and/or language services.

*(continues)*

**Figure 16-4** Caucuses and other resources for culturally and linguistically diverse students *(Source: Delmar/Cengage Learning.)*

- **Hispanic Caucus.** The Hispanic Caucus discusses and addresses problems related to professionals, students, and clients who are Hispanic.

- **Lesbian/Gay/Bisexual Audiologists and Speech–Language Pathologists.** The Lesbian/Gay/Bisexual Audiologists and Speech–Language Pathologists (L'GASP) group provides a forum to discuss issues related to L'GASP's professional needs and concerns, such as addressing homophobia in the workplace.

- **National Black Association for Speech–Language and Hearing.** The National Black Association for Speech–Language and Hearing (NBASLH) addresses the issues related to professionals, students, and clients who are African American.

- **Native American Caucus.** The Native American Caucus addresses issues related to clients and professionals who are Native American. The caucus promotes awareness of Native American culture.

**Figure 16-4** (*Continued*)

## CONCLUSION

Audiologists and speech–language pathologists from culturally and linguistically diverse backgrounds are in strong demand to meet the needs of a growing multicultural population of individuals seeking services for speech, language, and hearing disorders. For students from a culturally and linguistically diverse background, there are many resources available to help achieve success in their undergraduate and graduate programs. By developing your CSD skills so they incorporate multicultural and multilinguistic abilities, you will find yourself well positioned for a successful career once you are ready for the job market.

## REFERENCE

American Speech-Language-Hearing Association. (n.d.). *Omnibus survey: ASHA membership counts by race and ethnicity*. Retrieved July 17, 2004, from http://www.asha.org/members/research/reports/member-counts.htm.

# CHAPTER 17

## Advice for Students with an Undergraduate Degree in Another Discipline

### INTRODUCTION

It is not uncommon for students to enter a graduate communication sciences and disorders (CSD) program with an undergraduate degree in another discipline. Individuals who may have worked for several years in a different field often seek the CSD profession when making a career change. Many programs are very welcoming of students from different disciplines and backgrounds. In fact, if you have a degree in a related area (e.g., linguistics, education, Spanish), this makes you very enticing to graduate programs. Your unique perspective can aid in classroom discussions as well as in clinical work. Remember that you will probably have to take 1 year of undergraduate CSD courses before taking graduate-level courses. This chapter discusses other factors that you should consider. Figure 17-1 provides a checklist to track your progress.

### CONTACT THE COMMUNICATION SCIENCES AND DISORDERS DEPARTMENT OF YOUR PROSPECTIVE GRADUATE PROGRAM

Ask to speak with the director of graduate studies and the undergraduate advisor in CSD to find out what undergraduate requirements you will need to fulfill. Consider asking the following questions:

- What courses will I need to take to graduate?
- How many credit hours will I need to graduate?
- How long does it usually take to complete the prerequisite coursework?
- What courses are required for teacher certification? (If you are considering working in a school, your state may require that you complete a certain number of education courses.)
- Will I need to take the prerequisite courses before I apply to the graduate program?

| | |
|---|---|
| ☐ | Contact the communication sciences and disorders department of your prospective graduate program |
| ☐ | Ascertain the technical term your school uses for students in your position |
| ☐ | Take some undergraduate prerequisites before beginning your program |
| ☐ | Observe a professional in the field |
| ☐ | Expect to take one year to complete most of the undergraduate coursework |
| ☐ | Get to know other postbaccalaureates |
| ☐ | Learn good time management skills |
| ☐ | Make time for fun and relaxation |
| ☐ | Make time for sleep |
| ☐ | Limit outside work, if possible |
| ☐ | Talk with students taking junior- and senior-level classes |
| ☐ | Join National Student Speech Language Hearing Association |
| ☐ | Become involved with your local chapter of National Student Speech Language Hearing Association |
| ☐ | Identify the unique qualities that you bring to class |
| ☐ | When things get tough, remember your goals |

**Figure 17-1** Checklist for students with an undergraduate degree in another discipline *(Source: Delmar/Cengage Learning.)*

- Will I have a better chance of being admitted to the program if I have taken some of the prerequisite courses and demonstrated an ability to handle CSD coursework?
- Do I need to apply for the prerequisite courses?
- Whom do I contact to discuss what courses from my undergraduate transcript will transfer?
- When are courses typically scheduled (night, day, or weekend)?
- Are any of the courses offered online?

## ASCERTAIN THE TECHNICAL TERM YOUR SCHOOL USES FOR STUDENTS IN YOUR POSITION

Some schools use *postbaccalaureate, prerequisites,* or *deficiencies* when referring to students in a CSD graduate program with a different major. Although the terms are synonymous, you should use your program's jargon.

# TAKE SOME UNDERGRADUATE PREREQUISITES BEFORE BEGINNING YOUR PROGRAM

If possible, try to get a jump-start on undergraduate prerequisites during the summer before your first year in a graduate program. This step will help your transition to full-time CSD coursework and may lighten your class load. Find out if it is possible to take courses on campus from the program you plan to attend. You may also want to consider online courses, which give extra flexibility if you are working or caring for a family.

## OBSERVE A PROFESSIONAL IN THE FIELD

If you have not done so already, observing a professional audiologist or speech–language pathologist in a variety of settings will help you evaluate whether you can truly picture yourself working in this discipline. Contact your local hospital, rehabilitation center, school district, or other settings where speech–language pathologists and audiologists work and arrange to observe them in the field. Additionally, ask the clinical director at the program you plan to attend to refer you to a former post-bachelor student who you could observe and speak with about his or her academic experience. These hours are to help you learn more about the profession and are separate from American Speech–Language–Hearing Association's (ASHA) required observation hours; most programs require observations as requirements of specific classes.

## EXPECT TO TAKE ONE YEAR TO COMPLETE MOST OF THE UNDERGRADUATE COURSEWORK

Undergraduates who major in CSD usually take 2 years of courses within their major. It will most likely take you 1 year to take all the CSD prerequisites needed before you begin a graduate study.

## GET TO KNOW OTHER POSTBACCALAUREATES

Only prerequisite students know what it is truly like to take all of the required undergraduate CSD courses in 1 year. Prerequisite students have a special bond that only prerequisites can understand. Share your experiences with other prerequisites. Exchange stories about the career path you took, or almost took. Developing relationships with students who have similar interests can lead to a great support system of people to study, observe, and work on projects with; you may find these relationships follow you through your graduate work.

# LEARN GOOD TIME MANAGEMENT SKILLS

You will need to balance your time wisely to complete assignments on time and prepare for examinations. If you have been a procrastinator in the past, this is a great time to overcome that habit. If you need help developing time management skills, find out whether your school offers courses through a learning center or academic advising office. You can also search the library or a bookstore for resources.

# MAKE TIME FOR FUN AND RELAXATION

Even though you are busy with class, work, and, possibly, clinical work, you have to make room for downtime. At least once a week, do something that is fun or relaxing. Continue to be an active member of the community. Relax whenever you have the opportunity, especially over long weekends and spring break.

# MAKE TIME FOR SLEEP

Find a way to balance your study time and sleep schedule. Most people learn and function most efficiently when they are well rested. Make sleep a priority.

# LIMIT OUTSIDE WORK, IF POSSIBLE

Trying to balance a full-time course load, studying, a full-time job, personal/social time, and sleep is difficult—and for many it seems impossible. Understandably, you may need to work for financial reasons. If working while being a full-time student is too overwhelming, look into student loans and other financial assistance. If possible, try to work only part-time to make your schedule more manageable. If this is not possible, consider taking courses part-time if that is an option in your program.

# TALK WITH STUDENTS TAKING JUNIOR- AND SENIOR-LEVEL CLASSES

Ask undergraduate juniors and seniors in your classes what they think of the courses. For instance, ask the seniors for advice on some of the junior-level classes. They may have insight into classes or sections that were particularly useful or have recommendations about professors who are particularly strong instructors.

# JOIN NATIONAL STUDENT SPEECH LANGUAGE HEARING ASSOCIATION

Refer to Chapter 24 in this guide, or visit the National Student Speech Language Hearing Association (NSSLHA) Web site to learn more about the many benefits of joining the national association.

# BECOME INVOLVED WITH YOUR LOCAL CHAPTER OF NATIONAL STUDENT SPEECH LANGUAGE HEARING ASSOCIATION

Joining your local NSSLHA chapter is a great way to become an active member of your school's CSD community and to learn more about the profession. You can get to know your classmates at social events and become involved with volunteer activities.

# IDENTIFY THE UNIQUE QUALITIES THAT YOU BRING TO CLASS

It may be frustrating to have an undergraduate degree and still be taking undergraduate classes. Use your experience to help other students in your courses and enrich your own educational experience. The skills that you have gained from your first undergraduate degree can be put to use in CSD. For example, someone with a degree in special education is familiar with the Individuals with Disabilities Education Act (IDEA) and Individual Education Plans (IEPs) that are required by law and therefore can share those relevant experiences with the class.

# WHEN THINGS GET TOUGH, REMEMBER YOUR GOALS

Hard work in school will lead to greater payoffs in the future. Picture yourself as a successful clinician/scientist whenever you doubt your abilities or are feeling overwhelmed by the demands on your time. A positive attitude is the key to a promising future. If you are passionate about the field and believe in yourself, you will make it through.

# CONCLUSION

Students with majors in fields other than CSD can most certainly obtain a graduate degree in audiology or speech–language pathology, but the road to a successful career will be a little longer than for traditional CSD majors. However, you bring to your studies all the knowledge you gained from your first major, which can give you a valuable perspective on issues in CSD and may translate to an even more successful professional practice. Use this chapter to help identify actions you will need to take to get the most out of your prerequisite courses and to transition smoothly into graduate coursework.

# CHAPTER 18

# Advice for U.S. and International Students Studying Abroad

## INTRODUCTION

Colleges in the United States, Canada, Greece, and Saudi Arabia have National Student Speech Language Hearing Association (NSSLHA) chapters on their campuses. NSSLHA is receiving an ever-increasing number of questions from students abroad about programs and work requirements in the United States. The national office also is receiving questions from students in the United States who want to study abroad. This chapter will explain how to locate a communication sciences and disorders (CSD) program and what you need to know to study abroad. The first section of the chapter will focus on American students who want to study CSD internationally. The second half of the chapter will provide information to international students interested in studying in the United States. Each section will end with frequently asked questions (FAQs) from students. In this chapter, when we use the term *international*, unless otherwise stated, that includes students from Canada.

## INFORMATION FOR AMERICAN STUDENTS STUDYING ABROAD

As we become a more global-thinking population, the idea of studying internationally becomes appealing. Understanding how other cultures process language and norms makes for a more robust professional.

If you have an interest in learning in another country, there are several resources available on the Internet. (Search for "study communication sciences and disorders internationally" in any search engine.) Studyabroad.com is a Web site that offers a step-by-step handbook with tips for both students and their parents. Students may use this site to identify graduate and undergraduate CSD programs worldwide. Their Study Abroad Student Guide offers information on everything from how to obtain academic credit, to how to research study-abroad opportunities. Also, the U.S. Department of State's Web site provides details and advice on new requirements for travelers and the steps to register a visit abroad.

The FAQs below address other questions that American students have about studying abroad.

**Q. *Where can I find information about international training or volunteer opportunities on the American Speech–Language–Hearing Association (ASHA) Web site?***

**A.** ASHA's Office of Multicultural Affairs maintains a list of audiology and speech–language pathology organizations outside the United States. Contacting one of these organizations may assist in locating opportunities abroad.

**Q. *Can an American student complete master's coursework oversees and receive ASHA membership and certification?***

**A.** Applying for ASHA membership and certification after completing a graduate degree in another country would require you to have your credentials evaluated by a special evaluating agency and would require that your ASHA application be evaluated to determine that you have met the 2005 Certification Standards in Speech–Language Pathology or the 2007 Certification Standards in Audiology. Individuals applying for certification in speech–language pathology would still have to take the Praxis Series examination in speech–language pathology and complete a clinical fellowship, and applicants for certification in audiology would need to successfully complete the Praxis Series examination in audiology.

**Q. *I have seen mention of a Multilateral Mutual Recognition Agreement (MMRA)? What is this and how does it impact students?***

**A.** The Multilateral Mutual Recognition Agreement (or "the Agreement") is an arrangement between the ASHA (United States), the Canadian Association of Speech–Language Pathologists and Audiologists (CASLPA) (Canada), the Royal College of Speech and Language Therapists (United Kingdom), the Speech Pathology Association of Australia Limited (Australia), the Irish Association of Speech and Language Therapists (Ireland), and the New Zealand Speech–Language Therapists' Association (New Zealand) to mutually recognize the certification programs in speech–language pathology that they each conduct. There is no agreement for recognition in audiology, and the MMRA does not have an impact on students. It pertains only to those professionals who are already recognized by one of the signatory associations.

The ASHA Web site has complete information on the Agreement, along with application forms and a set of FAQs. Search the ASHA Web site for "membership and certification." Then search for "Multilateral Mutual Recognition Agreement."

**Q. *How does a student with an international degree apply for ASHA certification under the Agreement?***

**A.** If you complete your education and receive your degree outside the United States and wish to apply for ASHA certification without already having gained certification from one of the other signatory associations, you will need to apply to ASHA as a foreign applicant and will need to submit your educational transcripts to a foreign credential review agency for translation into the American semester hours system, for determining which courses were completed at the graduate level, and for a statement that the degree earned in the foreign institution is equivalent to a U.S. graduate degree. Please keep in mind that those individuals applying in audiology as of January 1, 2012, must have an earned doctoral degree.

You would then submit that information, along with a fully completed application for certification, your transcripts, and fees to ASHA for processing. ASHA would then evaluate your application to determine whether the requirements for approving academic coursework and clinical practicum are met. You would, of course, need to complete a supervised clinical fellowship experience and take and successfully complete the Praxis Series examination in speech–language pathology. The ASHA Web site has a listing of foreign credential review agencies. Search for "ASHA certification credential evaluation."

**Q.** *Can a professional certified by an international credentialing body supervise a clinical fellow from the United States?*

**A.** ASHA-certified individuals must supervise clinical practicum hours that will be used for ASHA certification. The Multilateral Mutual Recognition Agreement does not permit individuals certified outside the United States to supervise clinical practicum hours for students in U.S. programs. The Agreement does, however, permit you to do a clinical fellowship under the supervision of an individual holding either ASHA certification or CASLPA certification.

**Q.** *What do U.S. citizens need to do in order to work in another country?*

**A.** A U.S. citizen who wishes to work in a country in which he or she is not a citizen must meet that country's visa, work permit, education, licensing, and regulatory requirements. For additional information, please contact the embassy or consulate of the country in which you wish to work.

Note: The following commercial Web sites may be helpful when planning to work in another country:

www.embassyworld.com—for more information on embassies
http://projectvisa.com—for more information on visas
www.workpermit.com—for more information on work permits

(The inclusion of these Web sites does not imply their endorsement.)

ASHA's Web site has information about finding positions with U.S. agencies (e.g., uniformed services, federal government, or school systems) in other countries. Also, the site has a list of speech–language pathology and audiology associations in other countries. Search for "audiology and speech-language pathology associations outside of the United States."

American citizens interested in working in a country within the European Union should contact the Comité Permanent de Liaison des Orthophonistes/ Logopèdes de l'Union Européenne (CPLOL), or Standing Liaison Committee of Speech and Language Therapists/Logopedists in the European Union.

# INFORMATION FOR INTERNATIONAL STUDENTS

Studying in the United States is an opportunity for international students to experience CSD at the institutions responsible for founding the discipline. Fortunately, there are several resources on the Internet to guide students. Studyabroad.com is one such resource. It is a directory listing study-abroad programs, including summer study abroad, internship, service learning and volunteer abroad, high school study abroad, and intensive language programs—all by subject, country, or city. Moreover, choosing the course that best fits your future career goals can be challenging. ASHA's online, on-demand, academic program search engine, EDFIND is the most comprehensive database of all CSD programs in the United States. You can use this search engine to view and choose CSD programs by the area of study, location, financial support, distance education options, among others.

**Q. *What is the procedure for admission to an American school?***

**A.** Most college and university Web sites list their admission procedures. Follow the procedures mentioned in the program's admission process. For the most part, the process is the same as for an American student, except that there may be a few extra steps verifying coursework.

**Q. *Is the Graduate Record Examination (GRE) required to attend an American school?***

**A.** The answer depends on the school. Some schools require the GRE or an equivalent examination for entry. It is best to contact the admissions office and speak with someone knowledgeable about that school's requirements.

**Q. *Can students from outside the United States join the National Student Speech Language Hearing Association (NSSLHA) and receive benefits?***

**A.** Yes. NSSLHA membership is available to all students enrolled in a communication sciences program either in the United States or abroad.

**Q. *Will NSSLHA's liability insurance cover students coming to the United States to complete an internship or will the student receive coverage under the supervisor's liability coverage?***

**A.** Any student who joins NSSLHA is eligible to receive liability coverage through Marsh Insurance. Direct your specific questions about liability limits and types of coverage to Marsh Affinity Group Services. They can be reached by telephone at 1-800-503-9230.

It may also be possible that the student is covered by the supervising member's insurance. To be certain, have the supervisor contact the insurance provider.

**Q.** *Once in the United States, how can international students connect with other international students?*

**A.** International students can connect with one another through one of ASHA's Multicultural Constituency Groups. (See Figure 16.4 for a list of recognized constituency groups or caucuses.) All of the caucuses allow, in fact, encourage student membership, some at no cost. Also, Special Interest Division 14 focuses on communication disorders and sciences in culturally and linguistically diverse populations; therefore, joining this division will keep you connected with professionals and students interested in this area.

**Q.** *I plan to return to my country after I graduate from master's program. Will I need to take the Praxis Series examination?*

**A.** The Praxis Series examination is administered to students in the United States seeking certification to work in the country. International students who do not plan on working in the United States and who do not plan to pursue certification by ASHA need not take this test.

**Q.** *Is the reduced fee to attend the ASHA convention available to foreign students?*

**A.** Any student who meets the criteria for NSSLHA membership or ASHA's graduate student membership can avail of the discounted rate to attend the ASHA convention.

**Q.** *How does a student with certification from one of the associations in the Agreement apply for ASHA certification?*

**A.** The Multilateral Mutual Recognition Agreement (or "the Agreement") is an arrangement between the ASHA (United States), the Canadian Association of Speech–Language Pathologists and Audiologists (CASLPA) (Canada), the Royal College of Speech and Language Therapists (United Kingdom), the Speech Pathology Association of Australia Limited (Australia), the Irish Association of Speech and Language Therapists (Ireland), and the New Zealand Speech–Language Therapists' Association (New Zealand) to mutually recognize the certification programs in speech–language pathology that they each conduct.

Canadian professionals certified by CASLPA in speech–language pathology may apply for ASHA certification as a foreign applicant, submit a verification of CASLPA certification, and complete a 36-week clinical fellowship.

Professionals who are members of and certified by the other signatory associations can apply for ASHA certification in speech–language pathology. To be certified by ASHA, you need to obtain a letter of verification from the home association confirming current membership and that you are a certificate holder in good standing and need to submit an abbreviated certification application along with, of course, the letter and fees. Your academic coursework and clinical practicum need not be evaluated by a foreign credential review agency. You would, however, be required to take the Praxis Series examination in speech–language pathology and complete a clinical fellowship.

**Q. *Can a CASLPA-certified professional supervise a clinical fellow from the United States?***

**A.** As per the Agreement, only ASHA-certified individuals can supervise the clinical practicum hours that will be used for ASHA certification. The Agreement, however, does permit you to do a clinical fellowship under the supervision of an individual holding either ASHA or CASLPA certification.

**Q. *Is a degree in education and SLP (or something similar) needed to work in the United States?***

**A.** Each state has its own requirements for working. These requirements apply to anyone seeking employment as an audiologist or speech–language pathologist. To know the requirements of each state, contact the state audiology or speech–language pathology association where you are interested in working. You may find Web site links to all state speech and hearing associations on the ASHA Web site. Search for ASHA state by state.

**Q. *What is needed to work as a speech therapist in the United States?***

**A.** As an internationally educated speech–language pathologist, if you wish to become ASHA certified, you will first need to submit your transcripts to one of the foreign credential review agencies and will have to request the agency to provide you the following information: (1) a course-by-course translation of your education into the American semester hour system; (2) an indication as to which courses were taken at the graduate level; and (3) a statement indicating what your international degree is equivalent to in the United States, that is, whether your degree is equivalent to a U.S. bachelor's degree, a U.S. master's degree, or a U.S. doctoral degree? You would then be required to provide the information from the evaluating agency along with a completed application form and fees. When these are received, your coursework and clinical practicum will be evaluated to determine whether or not you have met the ASHA certification standards in effect at the time your application is submitted. Understand that the foreign credential review agency does not make this determination and that the agency's indication that you have a graduate degree does not imply that you will meet ASHA certification standards.

If you meet the academic coursework, clinical practicum, and knowledge and skills requirements for certification, you will need to complete a supervised clinical fellowship and take and pass the Praxis

Series examination in speech–language pathology; if you are applying for certification in audiology, you will just need to successfully complete the Praxis Series examination in audiology—audiology certification does not require completion of a clinical fellowship experience.

**Q.** *How can I learn about the logistics of working in the United States (i.e., green card, work visa, sponsorship to work in the United States)?*

**A.** The ASHA Web site has several articles on the subject matter. Search for "CSD Learning Abroad—Opportunities for All" by Michelle Ferketic, director, Special Interest Divisions and international liaison programs. Also search for working abroad tips, including job search resources.

**Q.** *How do I join ASHA as an International affiliate?*

**A.** *International Affiliate* membership in ASHA is open only to individuals who reside abroad and who are not exclusively citizens of the United States. Dual citizens may also become International Affiliates as long as they reside outside of the United States. You must hold a master's degree or the equivalent to be eligible and should be aware that International Affiliates are not eligible for and do not hold ASHA's Certificate of Clinical Competence. You must also agree to abide by an ethical code of professional practice statement that prohibits use of affiliation with the American Speech-Language-Hearing Association in the promotion of commercial products.

Individuals joining ASHA as *International Affiliates* are afforded limited benefits of membership. Please refer to the International Affiliate application for benefit information.

**Q.** *Will having a foreign dialect keep me from working?*

**A.** Students are encouraged to read a copy of ASHA's policy document "Students and Professionals Who Speak English with Accents and Nonstandard Dialects: Issues and Recommendations." The document should reassure you that qualified professionals should not have a problem seeking work.

## CONCLUSION

For students interested in expanding their breadth and depth of knowledge in the discipline, spending time abroad is a next logical step in their academic and professional development. The key to having a successful experience is to learn all the requirements for studying abroad and educating yourself about the requirements to work in any country upon your return.

# PART 4

# The Basics of Money, Research, Writing, and Interviews

# CHAPTER 19

# Financing Your Communication Sciences and Disorders Education

## INTRODUCTION

A college degree is likely one of the largest financial investments in a person's lifetime. Therefore, you could use some help to pay for your college education. Fortunately, the federal government, independent agencies, and educational institutions offer a wide range of financial-aid services and scholarship opportunities. This chapter provides some details on applying for federal student loans and obtaining scholarships and grants through American Speech–Language–Hearing Foundation (ASHFoundation) and other useful Web sites. The information contained in this chapter comes from the lessons learned by communication sciences and disorders (CSD) students in pursuit of funding.

## FINANCIAL AID THROUGH THE FEDERAL GOVERNMENT

The federal government is an excellent place to begin your search for college funding. Some students, however, dismiss this alternate as an option because they assume that only low-income students can seek federal assistance. It is true that students with greatest financial need benefit most from federal government resources; however, there are other federal government–sponsored financial-aid programs that support students at any income level. Figure 19-1 provides a checklist of key steps in applying for federal government–sponsored financial aid.

☐ Complete the Free Application for Federal Student Aid
☐ Apply for student loans
☐ Visit the financial-aid office at your college
☐ Keep copies of the financial-aid forms

**Figure 19-1** Obtaining federal government–sponsored financial aid *(Source: Delmar/ Cengage Learning.)*

# Complete the Free Application for Federal Student Aid

The Free Application for Federal Student Aid (FAFSA) is a report used by financial-aid offices of educational institutes to determine individual student eligibility for federal aid. The FAFSA Web site (fafsa.ed.gov) provides step-by-step instructions for completing the form.

You must file a FAFSA every year you are applying for financial aid. Applications for the new school year are available as early as July 1, and the federal government deadline for submitting the application is June 30. Deadlines for the FAFSA vary for different states, so refer to the schedule of deadlines listed on the FAFSA Web site or check with your financial-aid office.

Most financial aid is distributed on a first-come, first-served basis, so it is important to apply early. Do not let the fact that you do not have tax information readily available keep you from submitting an application. You can submit your application early by estimating financial information and returning later to officially complete the application when your tax documents are completed.

The most important step in completing the FAFSA is gathering your financial records. You should have your current tax return at hand. If you are claimed as a dependent on your parents' tax return, you will need your parents' tax return.

After you submit the FAFSA, you will receive a Student Aid Report (SAR). A copy of the SAR is sent to you and to the academic institutions that you requested to receive copies. As soon as you receive the SAR, you should review it and make any necessary corrections because the information contained here determines your eligibility for financial aid.

Although many state colleges use the FAFSA as the only application needed for student aid, be certain to check with your school financial-aid office to find out whether additional financial reporting applications are required.

# Apply for Student Loans

There are several federal government–sponsored and private student loan programs that enable a student to afford a college education, such as the Stafford loan, Perkins loan, PLUS Loan (loans for parents), and private student loans through Sallie Mae.

Stafford loans are government-sponsored low-interest loans available to most students, regardless of credit history (except those who are delinquent or in default on prior student loans). Perkins loans are government-sponsored loans available only in cases of exceptional financial need. Parental loans such as PLUS Loan are government-sponsored loans available to parents. Private student loans, or *signature loans*, are available to students who do not qualify for the Stafford or the Perkins loans, but still need additional money to cover college costs. The interest rates on private loans are usually higher than those on other government-sponsored student loans; moreover, private loans usually require a credit-worthy cosigner.

## Visit the Financial-Aid Office at Your College

By visiting your school's financial-aid office and making an appointment with a financial-aid advisor, you avoid confusion and frustration when completing financial-aid applications. Bring your completed FAFSA form or SAR and your IRS Form 1040 and W-2 forms (including your parents' if you are claimed as a dependent) to your appointment, along with a list of any questions you have. Do not let frustration discourage you! The financial-aid office is intended to help you with this often-confusing paperwork.

## Keep Copies of the Financial-Aid Forms

Keep copies of everything! Remember, you will be filling out a renewal FAFSA each year you apply for financial aid. Treat financial-aid documents as you would tax returns, or other important documents. Keep them in a safe place, and retain copies for at least as long as you will be paying on your loans.

## Weigh How Much You Need to Borrow

Obtaining loans enable you to pursue your educational goals, but loans have to be repaid! Borrow only what you need. Once you begin your professional career, make sure that you pay the loans. Late payments or defaulting on any loan will affect your credit rating; this could affect you when you look to buy a house or vehicle for years to come. Consider how long it will take you to pay back a loan. Ask yourself, "If I have to pay back $30,000 or $60,000, how long will it take if I have no other commitments? What if I buy a house in a few years, or need a new car? How much will I be able to pay back every month?" Consider what would happen if you have a baby and you want to stay home part-time or even full-time; how would you afford your loans? Based on the salaries in the region where you hope to work, find out how much you can expect to make. Find out what the average starting salary is, and not necessarily what the average salary is across all levels of experience; professionals who have worked for 20 years certainly make a lot more than those who are just starting out. Some people need to take 10 or 15 years to pay back loans. Therefore you should carefully consider how much you need to borrow and be creative in finding other ways to afford your education and living expenses.

## OBTAINING SCHOLARSHIPS AND GRANTS

Grants and scholarships are excellent sources of cash for college. The money is "gifted" to the student. It does not have to be paid back. The challenge with grants and scholarships, however, is the large amount of time spent researching, compiling documents, and completing applications. Obtaining grants and scholarships is not a process that you can do last minute, and you have to exercise patience and diligence to get it done. Figure 19-2 is a checklist of tips to obtaining grants and scholarships.

☐ Spend most of your time working on the essay

☐ Maintain a high grade point average

☐ Be involved in organizations and keep track of your achievements

☐ Build a good rapport with your professors

☐ Avoid scholarships from companies that charge application fees

☐ Ask for a list of scholarships at your financial-aid office

☐ Ask your academic advisor about department scholarships

☐ Build Relationships with Administrative People in the CSD Department and Financial-Aid Office

☐ Find out about available graduate assistantships

☐ Contact the financial-aid office for information on work-study positions

☐ Visit the American Speech–Language–Hearing Foundation Web site

☐ Visit other web sites for additional student loan and financial-aid resources

**Figure 19-2** Checklist for obtaining scholarships and grants *(Source: Delmar/ Cengage Learning.)*

## Spend Most of Your Time Working on the Essay

Many scholarships require candidates to submit an essay because the only way scholarship reviewers can get to know you is by reading your essay. In fact, scholarship reviewers favor applicants who exhibit strong writing skills.

Answer the specific question(s) asked. Do not go off on an unnecessary tangent. Pay attention to any formatting or style requirements. If the scholarship application requires a double-spaced, typed essay (they ordinarily do), do not hurt your chances by submitting a single-spaced, handwritten essay.

To check for grammatical errors and clarity in your essay, always have someone knowledgeable review your essay before submission. Your school's English department writing center or career planning and placement department is an excellent place to take your completed essay to have it reviewed. You can also seek out a trusted teacher, professor, or advisor. Remember! The essay is the reviewers' only contact with you. It is important that you make a good first impression.

## Maintain a High Grade Point Average

Many scholarships require the candidate to demonstrate academic achievement, usually determined by a high grade point average (GPA). A 3.0 versus a 3.5 can be the difference between thousands of dollars in financial assistance. Keep your GPA up by seeking help from your professors and peers, studying your notes regularly, taking a study skills course, reading your textbooks and completing homework assignments, attending classes, and forming study groups.

## Be Involved in Organizations and Keep Track of Your Achievements

Gain experience and knowledge in the field by joining academic, service, or community organizations such as National Student Speech Language Hearing Association (NSSLHA). In addition to rewarding academic and social experiences, being an active member of a student organization provides opportunities for participation, involvement, and resources (e.g., journals) that many scholarship committees take into consideration. Scholarship committees typically want to know if you have been awarded any special honors, such as the dean's list or awards through your department.

## Build a Good Rapport with Your Professors

Most scholarships require letters of recommendation from at least one professor in your field who can describe your work ethic and academic achievements. Get to know your professors by asking questions during lectures or make appointments to meet with them individually. Professors generally welcome inquiries from curious, interested students who take an active role in their education. Getting to know your professors not only helps you learn more but gives you the opportunity to locate mentors who may help you grow into a better student, clinician, teacher, or researcher.

Always ask your professor if he or she would be willing to write you a positive letter of recommendation. (You do not want to be taken by surprise by receiving a negative letter.) Give anyone writing a recommendation letter plenty of time to complete the letter; therefore, do not wait until the last minute! If someone has agreed to put the time and thought into writing a recommendation for you, it is a common courtesy to give him ample time to complete the letter.

Once a professor has agreed to provide a recommendation, you should give her the following in a neat packet (e.g., large envelope):

- A copy of the recommendation form or the writing prompt(s)
- An up-to-date résumé or list of activities
- A stamped and preaddressed envelope (if the letter needs to be mailed)
- A note (e.g., sticky note) to remind the professor of the due date and full name of the scholarship (which the professor will probably want to mention when writing the letter), and
- A personal note of thanks to your professor for taking the time to write the letter of recommendation

Once you hear about the scholarship (especially if you are the recipient), make sure you share the news with your professor.

# Avoid Scholarships from Companies That Charge Application Fees

Many students have reported receiving letters or e-mails from organizations that claim to help find scholarships for a fee. Without further investigation, it may be difficult to determine whether such organizations are credible. Therefore, before sending any such organization money, make sure you have conducted a thorough investigation. If you are unable to reach the organization to ask questions, or if the offer may seem too good to be true, walk away! As with any solicitation received via e-mail or the Internet, never provide any financial information without first verifying the legitimacy of the company.

## Ask for a List of Scholarships at Your Financial-Aid Office

Contact your financial-aid office for scholarship information pertinent to your school and your major. Often, private citizens or alumni have developed scholarship funds that are only available to students affiliated with their college or university. The financial-aid office usually administers those funds.

## Ask Your Academic Advisor About Department Scholarships

Your academic advisor is an excellent resource for current information about scholarships and awards offered through your school's CSD department. Often, alumni or former professors set up scholarships for individuals in a specific major. You should also check your department's Web site or ask the department chairperson about scholarship information.

## Build Relationships with Administrative People in the Communication Sciences and Disorders Department and Financial-Aid Office

Get to know the support staff in your department, as well as in the financial-aid office. Often, secretaries, administrative assistants, and other individuals who work in the department may have up-to-date information about scholarships, assistantships, and other opportunities. They are an invaluable resource.

## Find Out About Available Graduate Assistantships

Many universities rely on graduate students for assistance with research projects and undergraduate teaching positions. Depending on the university and the program, there may be a variety of graduate assistantships available (e.g., research, teaching, clinical, and project). In exchange for the graduate student's work, some assistantships offer a tuition waiver, monetary stipend, or in-state tuition.

# Contact the Financial-Aid Office for Information on Work-Study Positions

Often, a university offers a work-study program for both undergraduate and graduate students. Work-study positions involve working in an office or facility on campus. Try to locate a work-study position close to your area of professional interest. This will allow you to earn money and gain work experience.

# Visit the American Speech–Language–Hearing Foundation Web Site

ASHFoundation is the charitable organization that provides scholarships for CSD students. Most of the scholarships available through the ASHFoundation fund graduate-level research. The foundation currently offers the following student scholarships:

- **Graduate Student Scholarship.** Available to full-time CSD graduate students (master's and doctoral) who demonstrate "outstanding academic achievement." Award: $5,000
- **New Century Scholars Doctoral Scholarship.** Available to doctoral research students who will commit to working in higher education in CSD on attaining their doctoral degree. Award: $10,000
- **Minority Student Scholarship.** Available to racial/ethnic minority CSD students accepted into a CSD graduate program; must be a U.S. citizen. Award: $5,000
- **Student with a Disability Scholarship.** Available to full-time graduate CSD students with a disability who demonstrate academic achievement. Award: $5,000
- **International Student Scholarship.** Available to full-time international, minority graduate students studying CSD in the United States. Award: $5,000

# Visit Other Web Sites for Additional Student Loan and Financial-Aid Resources

The Web is a good source of information on student loans and financial aid. As with any Web browsing, the integrity and accuracy of the information obtained on a Web site should be taken into consideration. The following are additional Web sites with information about student loans and financial-aid resources:

- http://www.aessucess.org—American Education Services
- http://ombudsman.ed.gov—FSA Ombudsman
- http://www.privatestudentloans.com—Private Student Loans
- http://www.rspfunding.com—Reference Service Press
- http://www.salliemae.com—Sallie Mae

- http://www.staffordloan.com—Stafford Loan
- http://www.studentloannetwork.com—Student Loan Network
- http://www.upromise.com—Upromise
- http://www.ed.gov—U.S. Department of Education

## Additional Professional Association in Communication Sciences and Disorders for Scholarships and Grants

Many of the professional associations in CSD offer scholarships and grants for CSD students. For a listing of these associations, see Chapter 27. To find specific information on the scholarship and grants offered by each association, refer to the individual Web sites.

### Scholarships for Undergraduate Students

There are ample resources for graduate students in CSD, but there are not nearly as many resources for undergraduate students. The reason is that the master's degree is the entry-level degree to practice as a professional. The prevailing thought is that students at the undergraduate level are prone to change majors and not commit to an academic career in communication sciences.

In 2006, the NSSLHA executive council created a scholarship fund to support the financial needs of undergraduate students. The goal is to encourage continuing education in the field among juniors and seniors who demonstrate a commitment to the professions.

The American Speech–Language–Hearing Association (ASHA) foundation administers the NSSLHA Scholarship Fund. The fund is endowed by donations from ASHA's Special Interest Divisions (see Chapter 26), NSSLHA chapters, and individual donations from NSSLHA and ASHA members.

The NSSLHA Scholarship Fund is intended for undergraduate juniors or seniors and can be used to apply to graduate programs, attend national and state association conventions, conduct research, or support a student through a summer internship in the field. Only students with national membership will be considered.

For more information about the NSSLHA Scholarship Fund, visit ASHA the Web site.

### CONCLUSION

Although it does take some initiative on your part to seek out and apply for financial aid, the return on the investment of time and energy can be significant. Starting early, being organized, and following the information provided in this chapter should ensure that you are successful.

# CHAPTER 20

# Research Basics

## INTRODUCTION

As an undergraduate or as a graduate student, you have probably heard about the projected doctoral shortages nationwide. The "graying of CSD faculty" will soon lead to many unfilled Ph.D.-level positions as more faculty members retire. Therefore, the field needs new researchers to replace those who will retire. Providing tips that were developed following a discussion with Raymond D. Kent, professor at the University of Wisconsin–Madison and ASHA vice president for research and technology (2004–2006), this chapter will help you determine whether research is the right career path for you by showing you how to get involved in the research and how to be a successful researcher.

## GET INVOLVED WITH A RESEARCH PROJECT

Ask your professor what she is researching. If the project interests you, ask if she has any paying position for an assistant available. This option will simultaneously fund your education and help you learn about research. If there are no paying positions, ask if the professor could use volunteer assistance. The experience gained working with a seasoned professor on a topic that really interests you is priceless.

If there are no opportunities in a research project with a professor, consider creating your own small-scale case study design with one of your clients. Consult with your supervisor to determine an appropriate setup for your study. Consider ways to test the effectiveness of your treatment, or try a new approach to determine whether one approach yields greater results than another. Conducting a client-based research project will also help you understand and implement evidence-based practice with your clients.

## TAKE A COURSE IN RESEARCH

If your department offers a course in research, take it! If not, check for a discipline-wide research course.

## ATTEND SESSIONS ON RESEARCH

The American Speech–Language–Hearing Association (ASHA) convention offers various sessions related to research. Usually in spring, ASHA hosts a research conference on communication disorders. Moreover, some state conventions offer research sessions. By attending these sessions, you will see how different researchers formulate research questions, set up studies, and present their findings.

## KEEP TRACK OF POTENTIAL RESEARCH QUESTIONS THAT INTEREST YOU

When you take communication sciences and disorders (CSD) courses, make note of questions the professors or authors of your textbooks say have not been researched or have not been answered. A great way to keep track of research questions that interest you is to jot down those potential questions in a notebook whenever you come across them. Such notebooks will come in handy when you decide on your topic for writing a paper or organizing a proposal.

## READ JOURNAL ARTICLES OUTSIDE OF CLASS

Outside of class, read about areas that spark your interest. You can find research questions at the end of journal articles where the authors discuss further research questions that need to be answered. When you find a topic that interests you, try to work it into projects for your different graduate courses. The following is a list of journals that ASHA and National Student Speech Language Hearing Association (NSSLHA) publish:

- *American Journal of Audiology* (AJA)—ASHA
- *American Journal of Speech–Language Pathology* (AJSLP)—ASHA
- *Journal of Speech, Language, and Hearing Research* (JSLHR)—ASHA
- *Language, Speech, and Hearing Services in Schools* (LSHSS)—ASHA
- *Contemporary Issues in Communication Sciences and Disorders* (CICSD)—NSSLHA

Additional journal selections are available in Chapter 26.

## TAKE A GRANT WRITING COURSE

If a grant writing course is available at your university, take it! Doctoral programs will usually address grant writing within the department. The course typically explains how to choose human participants within the guidelines of the Institutional Review Board, ethics, funding agencies, and how to write the review of literature, procedures, and methods in detail within the page limits.

Researchers do not always use only one funding source. For instance, a researcher may get seed money from a smaller funding source, such as the March of Dimes, and later seek larger support from the National Institute on Deafness and Other Communication Disorders (NIDCD).

A grant writing course may also explain the process involved in approving a grant. Here is a brief overview of the grant review process at the National Institutes of Health (NIH), NIDCD, and National Institute of Child Health and

Human Development (NICHD). Once you submit your grant to one of the NIH study sessions that are offered three times per year, at least two reviewers read, discuss, and score your grant. The reviewers evaluate grants on a scale of 1 to 5: the lower the number, the better the score. If a grant has too many flaws, an "NS," or no score, is given. If the grant receives a 1 or a 2, an advisory council who approves funding reviews the grant. The council identifies grants that address areas related to human health that have been neglected. The advisory council that reviews CSD-related grants may consist of otolaryngologists, neuroscientists, biological scientists, psychologists, linguists, professionals in CSD, and some public members related to the professions.

## DEVELOP QUALITIES OF A GOOD RESEARCHER

Learn the qualities needed to be a good researcher, and develop them if you do not already possess them. The following is a list of qualities a researcher must possess:

- Creativity
- Commitment
- Tenacity
- Diligence
- Value interacting with others (e.g., at conferences)
- Enjoy publishing
- Love for knowledge
- Independent learning

## CHOOSE A JOURNAL FOR SUBMISSION

Once you complete writing your research, you need to choose a journal for submitting your paper. Your results and discussion sections can help you determine which outlet would be best suited to publish your research findings. Choose a journal based upon the audience of the journal. The goal is to have your research findings impact the largest number of clinicians and researchers who would benefit from your research findings. Remember, you can submit your research article to only one journal. It is unethical to have the same article published in two different journals.

## CONCLUSION

Research is the basis from which new assessments, diagnoses, and treatments are derived and is fundamentally important to the growth of knowledge about CSD. If research interests you, create your own opportunities at the graduate and postgraduate levels to hone your skills, perform valuable work, and share your findings with the community at large.

# CHAPTER 21

# Writing a Thesis

## INTRODUCTION

Writing a thesis is a great introduction to research and may assist you in deciding whether research is something you want to pursue as a career. Many master's students write a thesis because they plan to continue their education at the doctoral level. In many doctoral programs, students who did not write a master's thesis must complete one when they begin the doctoral program. Writing a thesis as a doctoral student prolongs the doctoral program. In other programs, however, students write a "pre-dissertation" regardless of writing a thesis, where students independently pilot research and publish the research in a peer-reviewed journal.

In some master's programs, the tract for writing a thesis is clear cut. For instance, the program may have a research methods course, where the thesis is explained and chapters of the thesis are written. For other master's programs, students learn about the thesis from their advisor or research mentor and then write it independently or take thesis credit hours. This chapter applies mainly to students whose graduate programs reflect the latter scenario.

Realize that writing a thesis may be the most challenging academic experience you will have to date. However, writing a thesis may be the most rewarding experience you will have as a master's student. This chapter offers advice as you work on your thesis. Figure 21-1 is a checklist you can use to track your progress.

## IDENTIFY A TOPIC AREA

Choose a topic based upon the area in communication sciences and disorders that interests you the most. At this point, you do not have to know the exact research question(s) you will address in your thesis; think general rather than specific. Your research mentor and committee (explained later in this chapter) will assist you with the exact research question(s) for your thesis. However, be certain about the area you want to study. You will be devoting at least a year of intense research to the topic. If you are not highly interested in a topic and choose one because an advisor tells you to do so, you will find it difficult to complete the thesis. Ask yourself:

- Why am I interested in this topic?
- Did this phenomenon affect a client or family member?
- Did I first become interested in this topic because of a class that I had?
- What aspects of this topic interest me the most?

- ☐    Identify a topic area
- ☐    Identify a mentor for your thesis
- ☐    Consider whether to interview your own participants or use previously collected data
- ☐    Complete and submit the human participants permission form
- ☐    Realize that it is unrealistic to complete a longitudinal study during your 2- to 3-year master's program
- ☐    Form a thesis committee
- ☐    Register for thesis credit each semester you work on your thesis
- ☐    Know and observe all thesis deadlines
- ☐    Consider taking a statistics course
- ☐    Review the literature on your topic
- ☐    Write the proposal for your thesis
- ☐    Find out what style you should use
- ☐    Submit your proposal to the thesis committee when it is complete
- ☐    Complete your thesis when your proposal is approved
- ☐    Defend your completed thesis
- ☐    Follow your university's requirements for having the thesis catalogued and bound
- ☐    Submit your research as a poster presentation or formal presentation
- ☐    Submit your thesis for publication

**Figure 21-1** Checklist for writing a thesis *(Source: Delmar/Cengage Learning.)*

- What do I need to learn about this topic before I choose to use it for my thesis?
- What experiences can I have now that would prepare me to research any topic?
- What research experiences or projects have I completed in my undergraduate coursework that may help me if I write my thesis on this topic?

## IDENTIFY A MENTOR FOR YOUR THESIS

Choose a mentor based upon a research area that interests you. Refer to the department Web page, ask classmates, and/or ask your advisor which professor in the department researches your topic area. Depending on your topic, you may find that no one in your department shares your interest. You may have to change your topic, or find a mentor whose research interests most closely match your own.

Once you find a professor who researches in your topic, make contact by telephone or e-mail. Inform the professor that you are interested in writing a thesis and would like to pursue a doctorate (if that is true). Request a meeting to learn more about the professor's research and discuss the possibility of writing your thesis on the topic.

## Prior to the Appointment with a Potential Research Mentor

- Prepare questions to ask the professor by looking up journal articles, textbooks, or textbook chapters that the professor has recently published on the topic. Reading the professor's work will give you a better understanding of what he or she does and allow you to ask the professor questions about the research (which makes you look well prepared).

- Have a general idea of the direction you would like to take your research. This may not be the direction you finally take, but the professor may have questions for you about your potential thesis. It will help the professor make an informed decision about working with you if you are able to articulate your area of interest.

## During the Appointment

- Ask the potential research mentor what he or she is currently researching.

- Consider asking if the professor has been a mentor to other students who have written a thesis.

- Inquire about thesis guidelines or a handbook that describes the entire process involved in writing a thesis in your department. It is very important that you become aware of your university and department requirements and timelines. Often, this information will also be available on your university's Web site.

- Ask what areas within your chosen topic you should research.

## During and After the Appointment

- Evaluate how well you think you would interact with the professor if you had to work together for at least the next year. Is he or she easy to talk to, knowledgeable about the topic, and available to be a research mentor? Has he or she ever chaired a thesis committee before?

- Ask if the professor would like to be your primary research mentor for your thesis, if it seems like a good match for you. Most students have difficulty identifying a specific question to research because they have not yet learned enough about the general topic to know what questions have not been investigated. Your mentor should be knowledgeable enough about the topic to help. In fact, you may be asked to take on a small part of a project that the professor is working on but does not have time to explore.

- If your areas of interest do not seem well suited, or if the professor does not have time to be an effective mentor, ask for suggestions of other professors in the department who may be a better fit for you and your project.

## CONSIDER WHETHER TO INTERVIEW YOUR OWN PARTICIPANTS OR USE PREVIOUSLY COLLECTED DATA

If you use data that has already been collected by another researcher (e.g., faculty member at your university or another university) as the basis for your thesis, you could save yourself months of valuable time. Although the choice is up to you, remember that you will most likely interview your own participants when you write your dissertation in a doctoral program.

If you choose to select your own participants, the first thing you have to do is find them. Ask your clinic director if he or she knows of eligible participants. You can also contact any support groups in your area, or you could contact clinical faculty or local clinicians. Realize that even finding two participants may be challenging and time consuming depending on your selection criteria. Thus, after your proposal has been approved, start searching for participants right away.

## COMPLETE AND SUBMIT THE HUMAN PARTICIPANTS PERMISSION FORM

If you plan to use your own participants, you must complete and submit the human participants permission form to the Institutional Review Board (IRB) to seek their approval, prior to contacting your participants. Ask your research mentor how and when to begin the process. It is your responsibility to complete the forms and turn them in on time. Find out the dates for when the IRB meets and when to submit papers. Some IRBs only meet once each month. Try to seek IRB approval several months before you plan on selecting participants. You may need to revise your thesis before the IRB will approve it. Seek advice from your research mentor because he or she has probably had a lot of experience in having projects approved by the IRB.

# REALIZE THAT IT IS UNREALISTIC TO COMPLETE A LONGITUDINAL STUDY DURING YOUR 2- TO 3-YEAR MASTER'S PROGRAM

Longitudinal studies collect data on participants over a period of years. Do not bite off more than you can chew with your first major research project. Planning a longitudinal study for your master's research project will not allow you time to discuss results in your thesis, and may lead to complications with passing or approving the thesis. It is possible this could hold up the completion of your master's program and delay your graduation. It may be best to save the longitudinal studies for your Ph.D. or later in your career.

## FORM A THESIS COMMITTEE

Most academic programs require a thesis committee. Your mentor will be the chair of the committee and should help you form this committee, which typically has two or three faculty members in your department. Sometimes, a professor from an outside department is asked to join the committee. Members should either be knowledgeable about the topic that you will research or have special expertise to contribute, such as statistical analysis. Some academic programs do not start the thesis process until the second year of study. If this is the case at your university, start developing good relationships with potential committee members early.

## REGISTER FOR THESIS CREDIT EACH SEMESTER YOU WORK ON YOUR THESIS

Some programs may require academic credit for work on a thesis. Ask your department chair or research mentor about registration requirements at your university.

## KNOW AND OBSERVE ALL THESIS DEADLINES

It is your responsibility to know and observe all deadlines and required paperwork associated with your thesis. It is up to you to schedule meetings, ensure that required forms are filed on time, and disseminate manuscripts to all committee members. Set realistic timelines. Realize that not everything will run smoothly, especially if you are conducting subject selection and participation. Have a contingency plan and be flexible.

## CONSIDER TAKING A STATISTICS COURSE

If you have not taken a statistics course yet, or if you would like to enhance your statistical skills, register for one. Having a good grasp on statistics will enhance your thesis experience right from the start. You will be required to take statistic courses as a doctoral student. Ask your research mentor if you should take a statistics course and what course is recommended.

## REVIEW THE LITERATURE ON YOUR TOPIC

If you are not efficient at finding journal articles through your university's library or Web site, go to the library on campus that is related to communication sciences and disorders (CSD), such as the health sciences or medical library, and ask a librarian to show you how to look up journal articles. Some universities offer one-time, noncredit, minicourses on researching journal articles—take advantage of these courses. Moreover, ask your mentor for recommendations on journal articles and textbook chapters you should read. If you find a great article or chapter on your topic, use the accompanying reference list or bibliography as a starting point for your research. These references may not be the most recent, but they can provide a solid foundation of understanding for your topic. It is helpful to keep a literature review notebook with copies of articles organized by date. Also consider creating a matrix to organize the main points of your articles. Possible headings for your matrix could include the following: title of article, authors, date, purpose of article, conclusions of the article, and a section for your comments. Also, consider each article you read according to the levels of evidence in evidence-based practice. Organizing your articles in this manner will give you a quick reference sheet to refer to as you begin writing the literature review section of your thesis.

## WRITE THE PROPOSAL FOR YOUR THESIS

Ask your research mentor when you should start the thesis proposal process. The proposal typically consists of the first three chapters of the thesis and includes the literature review, statement of the problem and research questions/hypotheses, and research methodology. However, many departments have slightly different formats for the proposal, so ask about your department's requirements.

Ask your advisor for previous thesis projects he or she has overseen. These will give you ideas for the general layout, grammar, literature review, and other formats that can help you get started. You may want to refer to the book *Dissertations and Theses from Start to Finish: Psychology and Related Fields* by John D. Cone and Sharon L. Foster (1993).

Know that your committee will read your proposal. It is your responsibility to prepare a proposal that is free from errors, including grammar, spelling, organization, and presentation or layout errors. Committee members should be able to devote themselves to the project's content and not be expected to do significant editing. Have a friend edit the proposal or consider contacting someone from the campus writing center for feedback.

# FIND OUT WHAT STYLE YOU SHOULD USE

In most CSD departments in the United States, the most recent edition of the *Publication Manual of the American Psychological Association* (APA) is used for style guidelines. The *APA Publications Manual* is a useful resource for learning the APA style. Find out what the preferred style for your program is and stick to it.

# SUBMIT YOUR PROPOSAL TO THE THESIS COMMITTEE WHEN IT IS COMPLETE

When you have completed your thesis proposal, submit it to your thesis committee. The committee will review your proposal and provide helpful feedback to make sure that you have a successful thesis experience. In many programs, there is a formal meeting during which you will orally "defend" your proposal. This means that you present a summary of your work and answer questions. You may be asked to leave the room while committee members vote on the proposal. The proposal may be approved at this time. Be ready for possible rewrites. Depending on your writing style and knowledge of what a thesis entails, you may be resubmitting your proposal several times.

# COMPLETE YOUR THESIS WHEN YOUR PROPOSAL IS APPROVED

Once your proposal is approved, do not wait to complete the thesis. Collect data, analyze results, and write the discussion chapters.

# DEFEND YOUR COMPLETED THESIS

When you have completed your thesis, you will most likely need to defend it to your thesis committee and possibly others, such as the department chair, faculty members, and students. Talk with your research mentor or advisor about this process so you will know what to expect. Know and follow any departmental or university-wide procedures for completing this step.

# FOLLOW YOUR UNIVERSITY'S REQUIREMENTS FOR HAVING THE THESIS CATALOGUED AND BOUND

Most universities permanently store a copy of every thesis in the library. Your university may have special requirements for how your thesis is presented, copied, and bound. Know and follow these requirements.

# SUBMIT YOUR RESEARCH AS A POSTER PRESENTATION OR FORMAL PRESENTATION

Now that you have completed your research and successfully defended it, share your work with others by presenting a poster presentation or formal presentation at a state or national convention. Many state associations encourage students to give poster presentations. Contact your state association to find out the deadline for submission and what is required. Deadlines for spring conventions may be due the summer prior to the convention. Applications for poster presentations for the American Speech–Language–Hearing Association (ASHA) convention are usually due in April. Check the ASHA Web site for more detailed instructions on how to apply for the Call for Papers (CFP).

# SUBMIT YOUR THESIS FOR PUBLICATION

Research finds have practical applications once they are shared with the professional community. Share your work with your colleagues by submitting it for publication in a scholarly journal. Since your research mentor typically puts a great deal of effort into helping you produce a quality thesis, you should be aware that it is customary, but not obligatory, to include him or her as a second author of any resulting publication or presentation.

National Student Speech Language Hearing Association's (NSSLHA) scholarly journal *Contemporary Issues in Communication Sciences and Disorders* (CICSD) accepts student papers for publication. Visit the publication page of the NSSLHA Web site to learn more about the procedures for submitting articles for publication. You will also find information on the CICSD Mentoring Program that will pair students and first-time authors with a research mentor who can assist with writing a paper for publication. NSSLHA awards an honorarium for student papers accepted for publication.

# CONCLUSION

If you chose to write a thesis, you will embark on what will likely be one of the more challenging and rewarding experiences of your academic career. It may be the only major research project you engage in if you go directly into clinical practice following graduation with your master's degree, or it may be just the start of a long career of professional research and publication. It is very important to remember that the practices outlined in this chapter cover only the general process for researching, writing, and defending a thesis. Check with your program for information on the process as it applies to you specifically, and then follow that procedure exactly. With all the incredible time, effort, thought, and writing you will be putting into this significant undertaking, you do not want to find your thesis (and possibly your graduation) is held up because of misfiled paperwork, improperly followed procedures, or some other clerical error.

# CHAPTER 22

# Writing for the Clinical Practicum

## INTRODUCTION

We often associate only therapy—face-to-face interactions with clients—with the primary responsibility of a professional speech–language pathologist. Although the therapy is important, clinical writing is equally important to a client's program. Once the semester is over, only clinical documentation and reports tell what took place during therapy—the amount of progress a client achieved, how quickly a client progressed toward a goal, the client's behavior/feelings, what did and did not work, what kinds of activities held the client's attention, what the client liked to talk about, among others.

The University of New Hampshire (UNH) has been studying clinical writing and clinical writing instruction since 1998. This research started when clinical faculty initiated collaboration with the Writing Across the Curriculum (WAC) program, which is devoted to supporting faculty in developing writing curriculum. This chapter emerges from observations of those aspects of clinical writing that students most often struggle with, as well as techniques used to support student writing. We begin by identifying rhetorical aspects of clinical writing, such as genre, stakes, audiences, and readability, and suggest strategies for using rhetorical awareness to facilitate the writing process.

This chapter focuses on clinical writing in speech–language pathology rather than audiology. There are several similarities in writing between each of these professions, however, depending on the clinical setting and genre. Some of the strategies described may be useful to audiology students, as well.

Aspects of writing clinical reports that are particularly difficult to negotiate, such as reporting "good news" and "bad news," handling background information, writing objectives, and ways to negotiate these aspects of writing, are discussed. The strategies offered may not be applicable to writing in every practicum setting. For example, we often suggest revising documents after receiving feedback from supervisors or peers. In some settings, however, deadlines are so tight that a long revision process is not possible. Hopefully, the suggested strategies can be adapted to fit different situations.

## CLINICAL REPORTS ARE IMPORTANT

As one of the main modes of communication between you and others involved in the client's treatment, such as parents, teachers, health care providers and care-takers, clinical writing plays a valuable role in supporting a client's treatment.

The reports we write educate others about what we are doing, what we have done, and ways others might support and supplement treatment. These reports also serve to prepare the next clinician, as the pieces you add to your client's chart provide information that is critical to developing a treatment plan that supports and builds upon the work already done.

Clinical writing is also important for you, both as a student and as a developing professional. Composing reports not only documents services but also affords you the opportunity to construct knowledge and apply what you are learning about the field and about your client into your clinic practice. The treatment plan is the place for you to think through the goals and the steps you will take to get there. The progress report gives you a space to pull together and reflect on a semester's worth of treatment and experiences. Many of the readers of your clinical writing will not meet you in person, so your writing serves as a way for you to begin to establish your professional identity. For these readers, you are your writing.

## CLINICAL GENRES

When you write for the clinical practicum, you will write in a variety of clinical genres, including both clinical documentation and clinical reports (Figure 22-1). Clinical documentation refers to shorter, more-routine writing, such as daily logs, lesson plans, attendance records, and subjective, objective, assessment, and plan (SOAP) notes (primarily used in a medical setting). Clinical reports are longer, more-detailed documents that may be sent to a variety of audiences. These reports include treatment plans, progress reports, and diagnostic reports. Each of these genres can vary in length, format, and appearance depending on the clinical setting. The clinical documentation and report writing that you learn during the on-campus practicum will not always directly transfer to writing for off-campus practicum settings. For example, the long, detailed treatment plan written for the on-campus practicum may not be appropriate in a school setting, where the Individualized Educational Program (IEP) serves the same purpose. As a student, you will need to investigate writing practices at each of your practicum settings. You may want to bring copies of clinical writing from your on-campus practicum to initial meetings with off-campus clinical supervisors to use as a prompt to discuss writing conventions at that setting.

## THE STAKES

WAC specialists talk about writing falling along a continuum of stakes, ranging from low stakes to high stakes, depending on the roles of the writing and the consequences or outcomes of the writing. Lesson plans may be considered lower stakes, as these documents have a limited audience and are not part of the client's permanent record. Daily notes and SOAP notes have slightly higher stakes, as other professionals and insurance companies may view them. Diagnostic and progress reports are considered high-stakes writing, as these reports can determine how well a teacher or parent supports and supplements a child's

| Genre | Description | Function |
|---|---|---|
| *Clinical Documentation* | | |
| Objectives (benchmarks, goals, and functional outcomes) | Specific goals around which treatment is based. The traditional form requires that the objectives be measurable and objective. Standard components are:<br>• *Skill:* the target behavior/competency<br>• *Conditions:* the situations and degree of support anticipated for the individual to successfully demonstrate the skill<br>• *Criteria:* a quantitative or qualitative means of tracking progress; the anticipated degree of success and independence the individual will achieve | • Identify areas of priority to be addressed in treatment<br>• Provide a vision for what is to be accomplished to improve the individual's communication skills<br>• Afford a means for measuring growth |
| Daily notes (lesson plans, SOAP notes, progress notes, consultation note, assessment/ treatment checklists) | A record of each treatment session. May take a variety of forms depending on the setting. These are very brief notations that basically document that the service was provided, along with some information on progress with respect to treatment goals | • Verifies that an individual received treatment<br>• Date is always required<br>• Time of day and length of session may also be mandated<br>• Tracks progress<br>• May include plans for the next session |
| *Clinical Report* | | |
| Annual treatment plans (Individualized Family Service Plan [IFSP] for early intervention, Individualized Educational Program [IEP] school age, and Individualized Service Plan [ISP] for adults) | A collaborative document that outlines an array of services and supports. Written for and by families with input from any relevant disciplines. Includes starting points and end points for intervention on a yearly basis | • Ensures that children and adults with disabilities will receive appropriate support services under guidelines established by federal law<br>• A type of contract that outlines individual's needs and how they will be addressed |

**Figure 22-1** Clinical genres *(Source: Delmar/Cengage Learning.)*

*(continues)*

| Genre | Description | Function |
|---|---|---|
| Insurance forms | Forms submitted to third-party payers. Generally include clients' personal data, as well as numerical codes for the type of problem and service, along with dates and times | • Allows for reimbursement for services |
| Daily records (attendance logs, clinical hours, and schedules) | These records document the amount of time the clinician and client spend in therapy and track appointments | • Verifies that services were provided and/or that clinical hours were earned<br>• Schedules allow for time management and reminders of appointments |
| Diagnostic report | When a client first comes to the clinic, his or her speech, language, and hearing are evaluated, and this document reports the evaluations. It could be written at any point in the semester and is often cowritten, as students mostly work in a team to conduct testing. The parts of the report include *background information* (about the client's medical and speech therapy history), *types of tests conducted, description of each test, results from each test, summary of the results, clinical impressions* (the clinician's observations during testing), and *recommendations for therapy based on the results* | • Confirms or rules out communication disorders, differences, or delays, to determine the severity of the problem and to make recommendations for services<br>• Provides baseline data for planning treatment |

*(Continues)*

| Treatment plan | Written during the first few weeks of the semester, this document contains the following sections: *background information* (about the client's medical and speech therapy history), *goals* (for speech therapy), *rationales* (reasons for choosing the goals), *level of performance at beginning of semester* (to serve as a baseline), *objectives* (a breakdown of each goal), *program steps* (a breakdown of the steps that will be taken to achieve an objective), and *approaches/procedures* (a description of the treatment techniques the clinician will use) | • Outlines the direction therapy will take that semester<br>• Is reviewed and signed by the student clinician, clinical supervisor, and client or client's guardian |
|---|---|---|
| Progress report | Written at the end of the semester, this document contains all the sections that the treatment plan used but now includes results of each objective, summary of all the results, clinical impressions (observations made by the clinician and others who communicate regularly with the client), and recommendations (whether or not therapy should continue, what to focus on during the next semester, whether more evaluation should take place, whether the client should get support from other professionals, such as audiologists or occupational therapists) | • Allows the clinician to review the progress with the client<br>• Provides a starting point for the next clinician<br>• Communicates results to multiple audiences |

**Figure 22-1** (*Continued*)

program, how the next clinician follows-up on the work you do this semester, and whether or not an insurance company covers expenses. The stakes are also, in part, determined by who the writer is. For example, though experienced speech–language pathologists may consider lesson plans as lower stakes, the stakes go up when student clinicians write them. Lesson plans serve as a means of communication between the student clinician and clinical supervisor and are essential to the therapy process. Similarly, though experienced speech–language pathologists may write lesson plans as a matter of routine, beginning student clinicians may spend several hours developing effective plans for their clients before each session (Russell, 1995).

The stakes are high, but there are ways to negotiate them. Each clinical report you compose may go through several drafts, and each draft presents an opportunity to receive feedback from your supervisor and other graduate students. This means that the pressure is off the early drafts, although you always need to edit your work before submitting it to your clinical supervisor. You use these drafts to take risks in your writing and try different ways of presenting and organizing information, and different ways of representing yourself and your client to multiple audiences. If deadlines limit your ability to follow these suggestions, you can still revise your work with a clinical supervisor or peers after you have submitted the report to a client or professionals. You will then be more proficient the next time you need to produce a similar piece of writing.

## AUDIENCES

We often think of audience as singular—as one entity—but the audience for clinical writing, especially clinical reports, is multiple. Your audience could include the client, the client's family, teachers, future clinicians, other rehabilitation therapists, health care providers, insurance companies, and the legal system. The audience also includes your supervisors and, if the client continues therapy after this semester, the next speech–language clinician and other members of the team. One of the challenges of clinical writing is negotiating the needs and sensitivities of each potential audience member—communicating all that you want to say, while using a level of discourse that is specific enough for the professionals in the audience and accessible enough for the clients and parents, who may be less familiar with the terminology.

There are several strategies you can use to negotiate audience. One is a prewriting technique. Before writing a document, such as a progress report (a genre where balancing audiences becomes particularly tricky because so many audiences are involved), you can list the members of the audience and then briefly freewrite (jot down notes) to each of these readers, saying exactly what you need this person to know. When you write the first draft of your report, refer to these freewrites to make sure you address all the points that you want to communicate.

Another technique is useful later in the writing process. Once you have a full draft, bring the draft to several readers who are similar to members of your audience. For instance, after removing identifying information, you could ask a person who is less familiar with communication sciences and disorders (CSD) (such as a writing center consultant) to read the report to see if all of the language is accessible. You could ask a person who has considerable expertise in clinical writing (such as a clinical supervisor) to read the report to see if the language is specific enough. You could ask fellow graduate students to read it to see what picture they get of the client and to determine whether they have a clear sense of how therapy would be continued next semester. These different sets of feedback can provide a fresh look at your writing through the eyes of your audience.

## READABILITY

Part of writing to an audience is making sure that the writing is reader friendly. Readers gravitate to writing that feels warm and personal. However, the voice you use should also retain a professional tone. You want your reader to see you as both a caring therapist and a competent, knowledgeable professional whom they can trust. You can create this perception by using the word *I* to refer to yourself, a pronoun that is more personal than *the clinician* and shows confidence on the part of the writer. Using *I* also grammatically requires the active voice rather than the passive voice, a move that helps to close the gap between the reader and the text. For example, rather than saying that a test "was administered," you can simply say, "I administered the test." However, the word *I* may not be appropriate for all sections of a report, such as in behavioral objectives. In diagnostic reports, the word *we* may be more appropriate when a team of two or more clinicians is completing the evaluation. Also, remember that there is controversy in the field about the use of *I*. The American Psychological Association (APA) now endorses the use of first-person pronouns in scientific writing. This endorsement has led to greater use in other forms of professional writing. We advise you to ask your on- and off-campus clinical supervisors about their perspective on this writing practice.

Creating a picture of who the client is as a person also makes clinical writing more reader friendly. You can use the client's name in place of "the client" to make the writing sound more personal. In sections of clinical writing that are more narrative, such as the background information and clinical impressions, you can describe the client's interests and behaviors. Remember that the representation you create of your client will serve as the first impression of this client for the next clinician, so these pieces of information are doubly important. The use of personal names and details varies from setting to setting. For example, in medical settings, it is generally more common to refer to *the patient* in clinical writing as opposed to using proper names, and there is less room for personal details.

Another part of readability is the way that writing looks on the page. The use of white space, bullets, tables, and paragraph length all affect the way a reader negotiates and decodes a text. You can enhance readability by breaking large chunks of prose into shorter paragraphs, using bullets to list information, and including tables to present quantitative information. Use these features to help a reader navigate your writing, and zone in on the important pieces of information. Be careful, though, not to sacrifice evaluative or interpretive statements in the name of conciseness. Lay readers rely on your interpretation of data; therefore, accompany your tables with explanations that help readers understand the data.

## "GOOD NEWS" AND "BAD NEWS"

Because student clinicians work closely with their clients and care about them, students sometimes have a difficult time delivering "bad news"—such as lack of progress, lack of an adequate support network for the client, or difficulty with a client's behavior during therapy. UNH noticed this challenge during writing conferences. The clinical supervisor or writing fellow would finish reading a truly glowing progress report and say to the student, "Wow—it sounds like everything went well." The student clinician would then talk about the not-so-good news. In addition, delivering "good news" in a progress report can be difficult. It is easy to become overly focused on the negatives and miss the small, but significant, increments of progress. These distortions of progress can result from being overly focused on a certain member of the audience, such as a young client's mother who has attended every therapy session, or the next clinician, who needs to be persuaded to follow the recommendations. The best strategy for making sure that the progress report reflects a client's progress is to conference with another student or clinical supervisor. Your reader could use a technique called *say back* (Elbow & Belanoff, 2000). After reading your progress report, readers share their overall impression from the report. You then have the opportunity to see if their impression matches what you wanted to convey. Your readers can also look to see if what you have reported in the various sections aligns with the recommendations. If the earlier sections are written in glowing terms, but are followed by an exhaustive list of recommendations (or if the opposite occurs), then a gap exists and you may want to consider revising.

## HANDLING BACKGROUND INFORMATION

Writing the background information section of the treatment plan and progress report can also be demanding. The challenge of writing this section was made apparent during a UNH practicum writing workshop. Students were asked to prepare for the workshop by analyzing the chart of one of their clients who had been coming to the clinic over a long period of time. During the workshop, several graduate students reported their surprise at the number of passages in recent documents that were copied word for word from earlier documents, particularly in the background information sections. This writing practice is not necessarily problematic in the way that other "copying" would be. Unlike other types of writing, clinical charts are collaboratively written, in that they are composed of writing by multiple authors. However, repeating passages from other clinical documents may not make the best impression on your readers, particularly those readers who have been reading reports from the clinic over many semesters. The background information section provides an opportunity to show your readers how well you know the client. To avoid repeating chunks of text verbatim from other reports, you could try a prewriting technique. After reading a chart, close it, put it away, and then jot down what you remember about the client. When writing the background information section, base your writing on these notes and only refer to the chart for specific information (i.e., doctors' names, dates).

This challenge of choosing what to omit when writing a background section is more applicable when the client has a thick chart (thus indicating that the client has been seen for services for a long time). Although condensing the history for ongoing clients has its own challenges, developing the history for a new client can be overwhelming. Rather than sorting through piles of information about the client, you are instead building a description from a variety of sources that may include a case history questionnaire, an initial interview, and referral forms. Once you write this description, you may need to step back and ask yourself if there are any gaps in your information. Do you need to know more about the client's medical condition? Do you understand why certain decisions were made by other professionals providing services? Do you have a clear sense of the client's communication ability? After writing a first draft of the background section, you may find yourself needing to ask the client and his or her team more questions and planning initial therapy sessions in such a way that will allow you to make additional observations to fill in any gaps.

## WRITING OBJECTIVES

Most forms of clinical writing reference goals and objectives either directly or indirectly. Setting treatment goals and writing specific objectives related to those goals form the crux of your clinical practice. Goals and objectives serve as a mutually agreed upon contract for the services you provide. They help you to narrow down and maintain your therapeutic focus. It is also important, however, to be mindful of the "big picture." You will need to regularly consider your client holistically in the context of a variety of his or her environments so that you do not lose sight of the broader communication skills and needs. For these reasons, it is especially important to formulate appropriate and reasonable objectives.

Your own developing philosophies about communication will be the guiding principles behind your intervention procedures. At times, you may feel that the objectives you develop may not directly reflect your personal hypotheses. It can be a challenge to reconcile a social/interactional view of communication intervention in situations where a behavioral objective format is required. One way to reconcile this is to provide a rationale for each objective, which in turn will help a reader understand how the objective relates to the ultimate communication goal. Another way to accomplish this is to make sure that your focus is on improving the client's ability to communicate effectively in real-life situations, as opposed to simply correcting or reducing a problem. It may be reassuring for you to recognize that although the required objective *format* may be behavioral in nature, your overall *approach* to treatment can be based on a social–communicative perspective.

Objectives may take alternate forms in different practicum settings. In a school setting, the goals and objectives are generally connected to the curriculum. In a medical setting, the focus of objectives is typically on achieving functional, daily-living outcomes. Do not hesitate to ask your supervisor how and why objectives may be written differently in each practicum experience you enter. This practice may help you begin to understand the expectations for the setting. You may also be able to obtain example goals and objectives used frequently at each site. In some cases, the objective may be fairly general— similar to a goal or benchmark, such as "Sam will improve his conversational skills." Other settings may require a more specific format, such as "Sam will increase his ability to initiate conversations." In other situations, you will need to develop a traditional behavioral objective that includes three components: (a) skill, (b) conditions, and (c) criteria—such as "Sam will be able to initiate a conversation with familiar partners at least three times per day in response to an expectant gaze." The traditional behavioral objective most clearly specifies what you expect an individual to achieve and is, therefore, useful as long as you keep sight of the ultimate communication goals.

Now, we turn to writing resources that you can seek to support your professional writing development.

## WRITING RESOURCES

### Sample Clinical Documents

In each practicum setting you work in, ask if you can read samples of what your supervisor considers effective clinical documents for that setting (while maintaining confidentiality). Try to collect samples from the range of clinical genres used at that setting. In each setting, you can explore how that setting or situation shapes writing conventions, the implications of clinical writing for particular audiences, and how writing styles vary across individual clinicians. Your program may also keep copies of effectively written clinical reports from their on-campus or affiliated clinics. By skimming though these samples, you can get a sense of the range of styles and formats available to you. You can see the choices other student clinicians have made when deciding how to portray their voice, how much information to include, how to translate jargon for a lay audience, and how to negotiate the needs, concerns, and sensitivities of various members of the audience.

### Conferences with Supervisors

Your supervisors are important writing resources, as they provide a professional audience for your reports. Because your supervisors sign their names to your reports, they are mutually invested in both the treatment you give your clients and the way your reports are written. Conferences with your supervisors give you an opportunity to develop the writing skills you need both as a graduate student and as a professional in your field. To save time during the conference, give your supervisor an annotated draft ahead of time. On this draft, highlight areas you would like the supervisor to focus on and jot down any questions you have in the margins. These notes will show the supervisor how you view your own writing and where you are in the drafting process.

## Clinical Report Revision Guide

The clinical report revision guide, a resource developed collaboratively by CSD clinical faculty and WAC faculty at the UNH, is included in Figure 22-2. UNH clinical supervisors use this guide to help students reflect on their clinical writing. It is included here because we have found that when students complete the guide before meeting with clinical faculty, their clinical writing is stronger, discussion on writing during the meeting is more focused, and students need to revise their clinical writing less often. The revision guide can also be an important tool to use during the writing process as a way to check your own work. Feel free to adapt this form to fit the criteria in your program.

## Your Fellow Graduate Students

Your fellow graduate students can be your best writing resources. Plan to write in a computer cluster or student lounge at the same time, so that you can ask each other questions as you write. See if other students are interested in forming a writing group. E-mail drafts to each other to get advice. Set up times to meet to exchange drafts. These meetings can work as mini-deadlines to motivate you to get a draft completed early.

## Writing Resources at Your College or University

Writing centers, available at many colleges and universities, offer free one-on-one conferences with students on their writing. Writing center consultants can offer you the perspective of a lay reader, a perspective that neither your clinical supervisor nor a fellow graduate student can offer. You may find this perspective particularly helpful when composing clinical reports, as opposed to clinical documentation. Remember to remove identifying information from documents before visiting the writing center. Writing centers also usually have writing guides and computer clusters available to students.

## Report Forms and Templates

Many programs provide their students with some sort of guide for writing clinical reports, such as treatment plans and progress reports. These guides range from skeletal outlines of a report's organization to more elaborately detailed

Name: _____     Date: _____

| Use this checklist as a guide for reviewing and editing your reports | Yes | No | Comments |
|---|---|---|---|
| As I was composing this report, I adjusted my writing with the intended audiences in mind by . . . | | | |
| I used specialized/technical language when appropriate. When I did so, I provided brief definitions, examples, or context. | | | |
| I reviewed this report to make sure that it is well organized and chronologically accurate. | | | |
| I eliminated unnecessary words and extraneous information. | | | |
| I used simple sentences when appropriate. | | | |
| I avoided excessive use of passive voice. | | | |
| I used first-person pronouns (*I*, *we*) only when appropriate. | | | |
| I proofread this report for spelling, grammar, and punctuation. | | | |
| I included phonetic symbols if needed. | | | |
| I shared this report with another person for feedback (while maintaining confidentiality)and discovered . . . | | | |
| I read this report aloud and noticed . . . | | | |
| I have adjusted identifying information and background sections to reflect any changes since the treatment plan by . . . | | | |
| I have adjusted the verb tense of each section as needed. | | | |

Which part of the report was easiest to write? Why?

_____

_____

Which part of the report was the most challenging to write? Why?

_____

_____

If I had more time, I would change/revise . . .

_____

_____

**Figure 22-2** UNH clinical report revision guide *(Source: Delmar/Cengage Learning.)*

descriptions of what information could be included in each section of a report. If these guides are available electronically, they can provide you with reusable formats for tables and examples of test descriptions that are easily understandable to a lay audience. Although these guides can be helpful, they can also be misleading, in that they imply that clinical writing is a simple process of filling in the blanks. Also, these guides can imply that clinical genres are inflexible— that the specifications of each section are set in stone. Be sure to ask your clinical supervisor questions about how each clinical genre can be adapted to fit the demands of specific writing situations and audiences.

## Saving Documents

As mentioned in the above paragraph, many clinical settings offer forms and templates electronically. If you are completing your documents using a computer, it is important to preserve confidentiality. Students may not be able to complete clinical writings during the hours offered by the clinical setting. Therefore, students may use their personal computer to complete their writing, in which case it is important to delete all biographical information about the client. You can then save documents to a USB flash drive or CD, transfer them to a computer at your clinical setting, and fill in the identifying information. This step ensures that client information remains confidential. Saving documents in a reliable place will also make it easier to modify writings following revisions done by supervisors or as the needs of the client change.

## Writing Guides

There are several writing guides available that focus on professional writing in CSD, such as *Report Writing for Speech–Language Pathologists and Audiologists*, 2nd edition, by M. Pannbacker, G. Middleton, G. T. Vekovius, and K. L. Sanders; *Survival Guide for the Beginning Speech–Language Clinician* by S. Moon Meyer; *Report Writing in the Field of Communication Disorders: A Handbook for Students and Clinicians*, 2nd edition, by K. Knepflar and E. May; and *A Coursebook on Scientific & Professional Writing for Speech–Language Pathology*, 4th edition, by M. N. Hegde. These guides provide writing techniques, sample reports, and grammar lessons.

## CONCLUSION

You will not learn everything about clinical writing during your graduate program. Learning professional writing is a lifelong process, as are many aspects of our professional work. It is this continual learning process that makes our role as therapists so satisfying. Your writing style will change and develop as you learn and grow as a clinician. You will continue to expand your expertise as you face new challenges, meet new clients, write in new genres, and are introduced to new ideas about human interaction and communication. As an integral part of client care, clinical writing makes a real difference in people's lives.

# REFERENCES

American Psychological Association. (2001). *Publication manual of the American Psychological Association* (5th ed.). Washington, DC: Author.

Elbow, P., & Belanoff, P. (2000). *Sharing and responding* (3rd ed.). Boston, MA: McGraw-Hill.

Hegde, M. N. (2010). *A coursebook on scientific & professional writing for speech–language pathology* (3rd ed.). Clifton Park, NY: Delmar Cengage Learning.

Knepflar, K., & May, E. (1992). *Report writing in the field of communication disorders* (2nd ed.). Rockville, MD: ASHA Publications.

Meyer, S. M. (1998). *Survival guide for the beginning speech–language clinician.* Gaithersburg, MD: Aspen Publishers, Inc.

Pannbacker, M., Middleton, G., Vekovius, G.T., and Sanders, K. L. (2001). *Report writing for speech–language pathologists and audiologists* (2nd ed.). Austin, TX: PRO-ED, Inc.

Russell, D. (1995). Activity theory and its implications for writing instruction. In J. Petraglia (Ed.), *Reconceiving writing: Rethinking writing instruction* (pp. 51–77). Mahwah, NJ: Erlbaum.

# CHAPTER 23

# Résumé and Interview Preparation

## INTRODUCTION

Now that you have mastered your academic coursework and will soon graduate, it is time to stake your claim in a professional position. This chapter provides an overview of what you need to know to get a job as an audiologist or a speech–language pathologist. It also provides many excellent resources such as sample letters, sample résumés, and other documents to use in your job search. Just as with applications to degree programs, the more research you do to find the right types of jobs, and the more preparation you put into your résumé, letters, and other materials, the greater your chances of getting the job that fulfills your personal aspirations.

## RÉSUMÉ WRITING

The résumé is intended to secure the interview, which in turn is intended to secure the position. A résumé should concisely highlight your career goals, educational background, work experiences, special skills, accomplishments, and activities in a manner that will market you effectively. For any employer, your résumé represents your organizational skills. Figures 23-1, 23-2, and 23-3 are three examples of formats to consider when preparing your résumé.

The following are the essential elements of any résumé.

### Header

To ensure that employers call, mail, or e-mail you with relative ease, put your name and contact details in the header of your résumé. In the contact details, also consider using a permanent address. Avoid listing a work telephone number because a potential employer will often find it awkward or difficult to contact you at a place of employment. Moreover, avoid listing e-mail address that does not sound professional; snuggly_wuggly@email.com or partymonster78@email.com really is not going to make a great first impression to a potential employer.

### Objective

Your career objective should be succinct. It should show career focus, possibly emphasizing a couple of your strongest skills. You can always change the objective to fit a particular position. Avoid using personal pronouns (*I*, *me*, and *my*).

**179**

**Kerry J. Doe**

123 State Road • Orland Park, Illinois 60462
(708) 555-1111 • kdoe@mailbox.com

## OBJECTIVE

To obtain a speech–language pathologist clinical fellowship position in an education cooperative.

## EDUCATION

*XYZ University—New Lenox, Illinois*
**Master of Science: Speech–Language Pathology**

Graduation Date: May 2003, GPA: 3.9/4.0

**Bachelor of Science: Speech–Language Pathology**

Graduation Date: May 2000, GPA: 3.8/4.0 (Magna Cum Laude)

## CERTIFICATION

- Illinois Type 03/09 Certificate in Speech and Language Pathology— May 2003

- Illinois Test of Certification for Speech and Language Impaired— April 2003

- National Examination of Speech–Language Pathology and Audiology— April 2003

## SKILLS

- Fluent in English and Polish languages, both verbal and written.

## PRESENTATIONS

"New Trends in Speech Therapy for the Adolescent Down Syndrome Client"

- PowerPoint presentation conducted at the Associated Colleges of the Chicagoland Area Conference, March 2002.

## RELEVANT EXPERIENCE

*Wainwright Elementary School—Minooka, Illinois*
**Speech–Language Pathology Assistant (8/00–5/01)**

- Provided one-on-one instruction to kindergarten students requiring speech and language therapy.

*(continues)*

**Figure 23-1** Résumé sample 1 *(Source: Delmar/Cengage Learning.)*

**Kerry J. Doe - page 2**

- Implemented therapies designed by the school's speech–language therapist.

- Contributed to planning sessions at multidisciplinary committee meetings.

## CLINICAL EXPERIENCE
*Green Point Elementary School—Palos Park, Illinois*
**Graduate Student Teacher (1/03–5/03)**

- Conducted assessments and developed individual education plans for students with communication deficiencies such as dysphagia, stuttering, language delays, and articulation and phonological disorders.

- Incorporated modern technologies to assist cross-categorical students with communication disorders.

- Met with family members to discuss clients' progress and to establish future goals and objectives.

- Participated in Student Services team meetings and multidisciplinary conferences to discuss caseloads.

- Conducted a seminar for classroom teachers on ways to detect possible speech-language disorders.

*Claybough Rehabilitation Center—Oak Lawn, Illinois*
**Graduate Practicum Hospital Clinician (8/02–12/02)**

- Performed evaluations and developed appropriate goals and objectives for elderly clients with communication disorders such as aphasia, right hemisphere dysfunction, and traumatic brain injury.

- Worked extensively with elderly dysphagia clients, including regulating diets to avoid aspiration.

- Collaborated with occupational and physical therapy teams to provide treatments for clients.

- Acquired comprehensive knowledge of videofluoroscopy assessment instrumentation.

**Figure 23-1** (*Continued*)

**Kerry J. Doe - page 3**

- Maintained accurate comprehensive records of clients' therapy sessions.

*Smith Speech and Language Clinic, XYZ University—New Lenox, Illinois*
**Graduate Student Clinician (8/01–5/02)**

- Conducted assessments and established appropriate therapies for children, ages 5–12, with a wide variety of communication disorders in articulation, language, auditory processing, and fluency.

- Convened with parents to discuss children's development and further therapy goals and objectives.

**Undergraduate Student Clinician (1/00–5/00)**

- Developed and implemented individual treatment plans for clients with communication disorders, including apraxia, language delays, and articulation and phonological disorders.

## HONORS

- Knudsen-Kempton Graduate Student Leadership Award, 2002

- Speech-Language Pathology Senior Student of the Year Award, 2000

## MEMBERSHIPS

- National Student Speech Language Hearing Association (NSSLHA)

- Illinois Speech-Language-Hearing Association (ISHA)

## ACTIVITIES
*Speech Club, XYZ University*

- Communications Chairperson, 2001–02

- Coordinated a mentoring program for undergraduate speech-language pathology majors.

**References Available Upon Request**

**Figure 23-1** *(Continued)*

**Kerry J. Doe**
123 State Road • Orland Park, Illinois 60462
(708) 555-1111 • kdoe@mailbox.com

## Objective

To obtain a speech-language pathologist clinical fellowship position in an education cooperative.

## Education

**XYZ University**, New Lenox, Illinois
Master of Science: *Speech-Language Pathology*
Graduation Date: May 2003, GPA: 3.9/4.0

Bachelor of Science: *Speech-Language Pathology*
Graduation Date: May 2000, GPA: 3.8/4.0 (Magna Cum Laude)

## Certification

Illinois Type 03/09 Certificate in Speech and Language Pathology —
  May 2003
Illinois Test of Certification for Speech and Language Impaired —
  April 2003
National Examination of Speech–Language Pathology and Audiology —
  April 2003

## Skills

Fluent in English and Polish languages, both verbal and written.

## Presentations

"New Trends in Speech Therapy for the Adolescent Down Syndrome Client"

- PowerPoint presentation conducted at the Associated Colleges of the Chicagoland Area Conference, March, 2002.

## Relevant Experience

**Wainwright Elementary School**, Minooka, Illinois
*Speech-Language Pathology Assistant* (8/00–5/01)

- Provided one-on-one instruction to kindergarten students requiring speech and language therapy.

- Implemented therapies designed by the school's speech–language therapist.

- Contributed to planning sessions at multidisciplinary committee meetings.

*(continues)*

**Figure 23-2** Résumé sample 2 *(Source: Delmar/Cengage Learning.)*

**Kerry J. Doe - page 2**

## Clinical Experience

**Green Point Elementary School,** Palos Park, Illinois
*Graduate Student Teacher* (1/03–5/03)

- Conducted assessments and developed individual education plans for students with communication deficiencies such as dysphagia, stuttering, language delays, and articulation and phonological disorders.

- Incorporated modern technologies to assist cross-categorical students with communication disorders.

- Met with family members to discuss clients' progress and to establish future goals and objectives.

- Participated in Student Services team meetings and multidisciplinary conferences to discuss caseloads.

- Conducted a seminar for classroom teachers on ways to detect possible speech–language disorders.

**Claybough Rehabilitation Center,** Oak Lawn, Illinois
*Graduate Practicum Hospital Clinician* (8/02–12/02)

- Performed evaluations and developed appropriate goals and objectives for elderly clients with communication disorders such as aphasia, right hemisphere dysfunction, and traumatic brain injury.

- Worked extensively with elderly dysphagia clients, including regulating diets to avoid aspiration.

- Collaborated with occupational and physical therapy teams to provide treatments for clients.

- Acquired comprehensive knowledge of videofluoroscopy assessment instrumentation.

- Maintained accurate comprehensive records of clients' therapy sessions.

**Smith Speech and Language Clinic, XYZ University,** New Lenox, Illinois
*Graduate Student Clinician* (8/01–5/02)

- Conducted assessments and established appropriate therapies for children, ages 5–12, with a wide variety of communication disorders in articulation, language, auditory processing, and fluency.

**Figure 23-2** (*Continued*)

**Kerry J. Doe - page 3**

- Convened with parents to discuss children's development and further therapy goals and objectives.

*Undergraduate Student Clinician* (1/00–5/00)
- Developed and implemented individual treatment plans for clients with communication disorders, including apraxia, language delays, and articulation and phonological disorders.

## Honors

Knudsen-Kempton Graduate Student Leadership Award, 2002
Speech–Language Pathology Senior Student of the Year Award, 2000

## Memberships

National Student Speech Language Hearing Association (NSSLHA)
Illinois Speech–Language–Hearing Association (ISHA)

## Activities

Speech Club, XYZ University

- Communications Chairperson, 2001–02

- Coordinated a mentoring program for undergraduate speech–language pathology majors.

**References Available Upon Request**

**Figure 23-2** (*Continued*)

**Kerry J. Doe**

123 State Road • Orland Park, Illinois 60462 • (708) 555-1111 • kdoe@mailbox.com

**OBJECTIVE**

To obtain a speech-language pathologist clinical fellowship position in an education cooperative.

**EDUCATION**

XYZ University—New Lenox, Illinois
**Master of Science: Speech–Language Pathology**
Graduation Date: May 2003, GPA: 3.9/4.0

**Bachelor of Science: Communication Sciences and Disorders**
Graduation Date: May 2000, GPA: 3.8/4.0 (Magna Cum Laude)

**CERTIFICATION**

Illinois Type 03/09 Certificate in Speech and Language Pathology—
    May 2003
Illinois Test of Certification for Speech and Language Impaired—April 2003
National Examination of Speech–Language Pathology and Audiology—
    April 2003

**MEMBERSHIPS**

National Student Speech Language Hearing Association (NSSLHA)
Illinois Speech–Language–Hearing Association (ISHA)

**RELEVANT EXPERIENCE**

*Wainwright Elementary School – Minooka, Illinois*
**Speech–Language Pathology Assistant** (8/00–5/01)

- Provided one-on-one instruction to kindergarten students requiring speech and language therapy.

- Implemented therapies designed by the school's speech–language therapist.

- Contributed to planning sessions at multidisciplinary committee meetings.

**CLINICAL EXPERIENCE**

*Green Point Elementary School—Palos Park, Illinois*
**Graduate Student Teacher** (1/03–5/03)

- Conducted assessments and developed individual education plans for students with communication deficiencies such as dysphagia, stuttering, language delays, and articulation and phonological disorders.

*(continues)*

**Figure 23-3** Résumé sample 3 *(Source: Delmar/Cengage Learning.)*

**Kerry J. Doe - page 2**

- Incorporated modern technologies to assist cross-categorical students with communication disorders.

- Met with family members to discuss clients' progress and to establish future goals and objectives.

- Participated in Student Services team meetings and multidisciplinary conferences to discuss caseloads.

- Conducted a seminar for classroom teachers on ways to detect possible speech–language disorders.

*Claybough Rehabilitation Center—Oak Lawn, Illinois*
**Graduate Practicum Hospital Clinician** (8/02–12/02)

- Performed evaluations and developed appropriate goals and objectives for elderly clients with communication disorders such as aphasia, right hemisphere dysfunction, and traumatic brain injury.

- Worked extensively with elderly dysphagia clients, including regulating diets to avoid aspiration.

- Collaborated with occupational and physical therapy teams to provide treatments for clients.

- Acquired comprehensive knowledge of videofluoroscopy assessment instrumentation.

- Maintained accurate comprehensive records of clients' therapy sessions.

*Smith Speech and Language Clinic, XYZ University—New Lenox, Illinois*
**Graduate Student Clinician** (8/01–5/02)

- Conducted assessments and established appropriate therapies for children, ages 5–12, with a wide variety of communication disorders in articulation, language, auditory processing, and fluency.

- Convened with parents to discuss children's development and further therapy goals and objectives.

**Undergraduate Student Clinician** (1/00–5/00)

- Developed and implemented individual treatment plans for clients with communication disorders, including apraxia, language delays, and articulation and phonological disorders.

**References Available Upon Request**

**Figure 23-3** (*Continued*)

Listing an objective is important for résumés of individuals who may not have much professional work experience. You may, however, notice that individuals who have been working for a long time delete this feature. Until you have many years of professional experience under your belt, the objective is important to your résumé.

## Education

List only your college/graduate education, placing your most recent school first and working backward chronologically. Include any degree earned, major, minor, and graduation date. Listing your grade point average (GPA) is optional. Also, indicate the kind of maximum grading your institution used. Before you make the decision to add your GPA, consider that some employers have a bias against candidates who do not have a 4.0. On the other hand, employers may bias against students with a 4.0; they prefer a "well rounded" employee. Because your transcript will accompany the application, it is maybe best not to create an opportunity for bias before the employer reads the body of the résumé. Ultimately, whether you add your GPA on your resume or not is your decision.

## Certifications

List any certifications that you have attained, as well as licensing examinations that you are scheduled to take. You may mention the dates associated with those items.

## Honors

Indicate any scholarships, awards, or honors earned during your college career, including special graduation honors, membership to any honor societies, or awards such as dean's list.

## Activities

These are good indicators of your leadership skills, professional interests, contributions, and social skills. Include those affiliations of which you are or were a member at school and/or in your community. List the offices that you held with those organizations. If applicable, mention highlights of accomplishments that you have achieved in those organizations. If you prefer, you may list the dates that you were associated with those activities. Avoid listing those associations that have a radical or harsh political or social tone to them, because prospective employers may perceive that you have extreme, inflexible convictions. Often, employers are looking to get a picture of you as a person, and the activities you list are one way they get to know "who" you are. Also, do not forget to include professional workshops or conventions attended. Some employers value continued education beyond the academic curriculum.

# Presentations

List any out-of-class presentations that you have conducted, including where and when they were performed. This section is where you would list any poster sessions or other presentations at conferences, such as the annual American Speech–Language–Hearing Association (ASHA) convention. Use a standard style of reporting this information, such as that recommended by *Publication Manual of the American Psychological Association*—such styling adds a professional look and represents your knowledge of how to reference material.

# Skills

Mention any special abilities that you possess, such as computer proficiencies, instrumentation competencies, or foreign-language fluencies.

# Experience

Include your full-time jobs, part-time jobs, cooperative education, internships, volunteer jobs, clinicals, practicums, field experiences, and so on. List organization names, cities, states, dates of employment, job titles, responsibilities, and accomplishments. Use action words to describe your responsibilities and achievements, and be cautious to use the correct verb tense. Create phrases that are brief, but make them meaningful and at least five words long. List items that highlight relevant skills, special training, high-level accountability, and achievement. If applicable, mention quantitative illustrations of contributions and accomplishments. When listing your responsibilities, use aligned bullet points instead of a paragraph format; however, exercise caution when you use bullet points because sometimes they can make for a very busy page that is not easy to read.

The résumé should represent your organizational skills and writing style. The key is to be consistent in style throughout the document. When listing your experience, list the field placements before clinical experiences. Then put your clinical training experiences in an order that represents the type of position you are looking for. If your experience is in a hospital setting, then place the hospital experience(s) first. In addition, the primary experiences (or the ones that speak of the employment preference) need to be on the first page, so that the employer can see, in a quick glance, that you are a potential hire. The second page can list the previous job experiences; however, only list those that have some relevance to the skills needed to be an audiologist or a speech–language pathologist. Do not include retail positions or positions not related to the job that you are applying for in the résumé.

# References

A simple overall statement will suffice (e.g., "References available upon request"). However, you should probably have a set of references ready on a separate page, in case they are requested. You should have at least three professional references that speak of your work ethic objectively, such as current or former supervisors or instructors. It is common courtesy to ask permission before listing someone as a reference. You should also confirm that they are willing to write a positive reference about you. List names, job titles, company names, addresses, telephone numbers, and e-mail addresses. Figure 23-4 is an example of a standard reference page.

## Miscellaneous

Typically, the résumé should not exceed two pages, but it may be best to limit your résumé to one page. When deciding the maximum length of your résumé, consider the job setting you are applying for and how many applicants will probably be applying for the job. If you need to include additional information not applicable to any of the previous mentioned sections above, you may choose such heading as "Clinical Experiences," "Publications," "Licenses," "Additional Training," and "Professional Development."

Finally, arrange sections in the order that markets you best, with your greatest selling points ideally in the upper two-thirds of the document. Make certain that your section headings are distinct. Use italics, boldface, and bullets to add variety and to place emphasis, but do not overuse them to the point that your résumé looks too busy. Keep the content and formatting consistent. Use page margins of about 0.4–0.5 in. for the top and bottom, with 0.7–1.0 in. for the left and right. For ease of readability, always use an 11- or 12-point font size and a basic font type. Print your résumé on high-quality paper of a neutral color, such as light gray or cream. An employer typically reviews a résumé initially for only a minute or two, so it is important to thoroughly sell your skills and experience in a succinct way.

Always proofread (repeatedly!) your résumé to ensure accuracy and consistency. Have a friend proofread for grammar, punctuation, and consistency in your spacing around bullets or other features of your résumé. Make sure that if you use a period after one description of a job, you use a period after every description of a job. Employers really do weed out undesirable candidates based on mistakes on the résumé.

## GUIDELINES FOR WRITING COVER LETTERS

A cover letter is the professional letter that accompanies your résumé and can also be called *an application letter* or *letter of interest.* This section discusses the requirements for a cover letter.

## Format

A professionally styled cover letter utilizes a block format to give it a clean appearance. All the sections should be typed in single-space format, with double spacing used only to separate the sections. Figure 23-5 is an example of a common format used for cover letters.

**Kerry J. Doe**
123 State Road • Orland Park, Illinois 60462
(708) 555-1111 • kdoe@mailbox.com

## References

**Mary Jones**
*Speech Pathologist/Clinical Supervisor*
Harrison Elementary School
579 W. Main Street
Mokena, IL 60448
(708) 555-7777
mjones@dist157.org

**James Meyer**
*Audiology Professor*
ABC University
1 E. Wire Drive
Frankfort, IL 60423
(815) 555-2222
jmeyer@abcuniv.edu

**John Smith**
*Speech-Language Pathology Professor*
ABC University
1 E. Wire Drive
Frankfort, IL 60423
(815) 555-3333
jsmith@abcuniv.edu

**Patricia Washington**
*Audiology Professor*
ABC University
1 E. Wire Drive
Frankfort, IL 60423
(815) 555-4444
pwashington@abcuniv.edu

**Michael Williams**
*Special Education Resource Teacher*
Harrison Elementary School
579 W. Main Street
Mokena, IL 60448
(708) 555-8888
mwilliams@dist157.org

**Figure 23-4** An example of a standard reference page *(Source: Delmar/Cengage Learning.)*

**Kerry J. Doe**

123 State Road • Orland Park, Illinois 60462 • (708) 555-1111 • kdoe@mailbox.com

May 29, 2004

Melissa Smith
Assistant Superintendent
Fairview School District 123
7890 W. Main Street
Fairview, IL 61432

Dear Ms. Smith:

Please accept the enclosed résumé in consideration for the Speech Therapist-Clinical Fellowship position that is currently advertised on your Web site. I recently completed my graduate studies and I am eager to start my career with your school district.

In addition to a master's degree in speech–language pathology and its accompanying clinical experiences, my background includes a year of **experience as a Speech Assistant** in an educational setting. All of those endeavors have allowed me to work with a wide range of clients, assessment tools, and therapies. They have also greatly enhanced my **analytical** and **goal setting skills**, and have significantly increased my awareness of the qualities necessary to be a successful speech therapist. My **creative** and **enthusiastic approach** to instruction enables me to quickly secure clients' interest, which allows me to provide for a positive learning experience. In addition, my effective **listening** and **communication skills**, along with my strong sense of patience, tend to gain clients' trust in my commitment to their well-being. Furthermore, my solid qualities of **resourcefulness** and **perseverance** help me to earn respect from clients and colleagues alike. Thus, my experience and personal characteristics seem to make me a suitable match for a career in speech-language pathology.

I would appreciate the opportunity to meet with you to discuss my qualifications in detail. Please send me any materials needed to complete the application process. If you have any questions or wish to arrange an interview, please feel free to contact me at your convenience at (708) 555-1111. Thank you very much for your valuable time and consideration.

Sincerely,

*Kerry Doe*

Kerry Doe

**Figure 23-5** Cover letter example *(Source: Delmar/Cengage Learning.)*

# Header

The header should list your address, telephone number, and the date. The next section includes the recruiter's name, his or her job title, the organization's name, and its address. The salutation should be formal and directed to a specific individual, whenever possible. If you do not know whom to address the salutation, call and ask whom you should specifically address the cover letter to. If there is no way of ascertaining a specific addressee, then use the greeting "Dear Administrator," "Dear Employer," or "Dear Recruiter," *not* "Dear Madam or Sir" or "To Whom It May Concern."

# Opening Paragraph

Name the specific position or type of work for which you are applying and indicate from which resource (Web site, career center, newspaper, employee, instructor, etc.) you learned of the opening or organization.

# Middle Paragraph(s)

Indicate the reasons you are interested in and qualified for the position. Explain how your skills, academic background, work experiences, practicums, clinicals, internships, cooperative education, and activities make you a well-suited candidate for the position. Refer to the specific achievements or unique qualifications you acquired in those experiences. Review the requirements for the position, and then try to match them with concrete examples that prove you actually possess those skills. Mention something about the organization that motivates you to want to work for it. Avoid repeating the same information the reader will find on your résumé.

# Closing Paragraph

State your desire for a personal interview. Repeat your telephone number and e-mail address, and offer any assistance to help in a speedy response. Finally, finish with a statement that will encourage a response, such as "I look forward to hearing from you" or "I look forward to speaking with you further about my qualifications."

# Ending

The ending should simply read "Sincerely" or "Yours truly," with your name typed three or four lines down to allow ample space for your signature above it.

# Miscellaneous

Limit your cover letter to one page. Although it is all right to use the personal pronoun *I*, avoid using it too frequently. While still sounding professional and somewhat formal, try to use common language to sound natural. Review the letter carefully, because the reader will probably perceive it to be an example of your written communication skills. Print it on the same type of paper that you use for your résumé.

Just as you proofread your résumé, proofread your cover letter. A prospective employer may not even bother to read your résumé if your cover letter has errors. Consider asking a friend to look it over for punctuation and spelling mistakes, as well as clarity and readability. Your cover letter is your prospective employer's first glimpse of who you are. An unprofessional cover letter may mean it is also the last.

## INTERVIEW SKILLS

In an interview, an employer is ultimately looking to determine whether or not you have the necessary skills and experience to fill the position, as well as the type of personality that will connect with others affiliated with the organization. The following steps will help you prepare for the interview process.

### Before the Interview

"[E]mployers want workers who know how to speak, listen, and think effectively; who work well with people from diverse backgrounds; and who can make good decisions on their own and in groups."

—*Seiler and Beall (2000)*

---

**Top 10 Qualities that Employers Seek**

1. Communication skills
2. Honesty/integrity
3. Teamwork skills
4. Interpersonal skills
5. Strong work ethic
6. Motivation/initiative
7. Flexibility/adaptability
8. Analytical skills
9. Computer skills
10. Organizational skills

*Source:* National Association of Colleges and Employers, 2003

---

Prepare a brief statement (30 sec) that will tell the interviewer a little about you. Become familiar with what employers typically look for and consider examples that will address these.

***Do a Self-Assessment.*** Determine your short- and long-range career goals. Identify your skills, abilities, personal qualities, strengths, weaknesses, values, and interests. Determine how they fit the position for which you are applying.

Be able to cite concrete examples of how you have demonstrated all those intangibles. Use your experiences from classes, internships, extracurricular activities, volunteer experiences, and work experiences to extract those examples. Focus on your accomplishments whenever possible. Be prepared to explain the rewards and satisfactions of your career field that caused you to choose it. Recruiters tend to shy away from candidates who have merely stumbled into their profession without much thought.

**Research the Organization.** It is essential to know some detailed information about the company and the position before the interview. An interviewer may be reluctant to consider a candidate who does not commit time to previewing the organization or the position. Organization research also helps you to devise insightful responses and thought-provoking questions for an interview. Research the organization's mission, products and services, target markets, competitors, business strategies, plans, challenges, and factors and trends affecting the industry. You can obtain this information through the Internet, libraries, chambers of commerce, directories, and so on.

**Dress Professionally.** The first impression that you make on an interviewer is your personal appearance. Improper attire can distract the interviewer from anything positive that you convey about yourself during the interview. A traditional, conservative look is usually your safest bet.

*Wardrobe Suggestions for Women:* Pantsuits or skirt suits with hemlines that fall just below the knee are preferred. A navy blue, gray, or charcoal suit with a white, long-sleeved, cotton or silk blouse is recommended. Shoes should be black, brown, or navy, with a heel height that is comfortable for walking. Hosiery should be a neutral shade. Jewelry should be limited to one pair of simple earrings, a necklace, watch, and wedding band. Remove all piercing that might appear unprofessional to employers. Hairstyle should look controlled. Makeup should achieve a natural look, and nail polish should be conservative and neat. Avoid overwhelming perfumes. Keep all tattoos covered, if possible.

*Wardrobe Suggestions for Men:* A two-piece, single-breasted navy blue, gray, or charcoal suit with a white, cotton, long-sleeved shirt is preferred. The tie should complement the suit and should not be too "loud." Shoes should be black or brown leather and polished, with socks that complement the suit. Jewelry should be limited to a wedding band and a watch, and all piercings should be removed. Hair should be well groomed, and facial hair should be trimmed neatly. Avoid overbearing cologne or aftershave. Keep all tattoos covered, if possible.

**Be Organized.** You should arrive at least 15 to 20 minutes before the scheduled interview time. Allot yourself plenty of time to accommodate for getting lost, being stalled by construction, getting stuck in traffic, or having difficulty finding a parking space or the interview room. If necessary, consult an online map to gauge the distance and directions to your destination. You may be required to fill out an application before the interview, so bring addresses and telephone numbers of previous employers, professional references, and personal references. Bring extra copies of your résumé. Carry all those materials in a vinyl- or leather-bound folder, along with a couple of pens. Be courteous to everybody at the facility, regardless of his or her relationship to your interview.

## During the Interview

***Prepare for Both Traditional and Behavior-Based Questions.*** Some recruiters use the traditional method, in which they ask about your opinions and experiences on certain work-related issues. Others use the behavior-based format, in which they question you about past situations and what you did under those conditions. The premise of the latter is that your past actions may be indicators of your future behaviors. Be ready to discuss the kinds of leadership, teamwork, initiative, planning, and organization you demonstrated for a given situation. Talk about the scenario, your course of action, the result, and what you learned from the experience. If a question initially sounds difficult, take a minute to formulate the answer. Beware of "hardening of the categories." You may be asked about a client or specific disorder that you have not experienced, but if you consider the basic issues with the disorder, that is, neuromotor pathways, brain function, development of speech/language, you will be able to demonstrate your ability to critically think through the problem.

It is okay if you do not know specifics about a particular client or disorder as long as you express how you would go about learning the specifics of a client or disorder. Whether you are familiar with a specific disorder or not, demonstrate that you know what resources to utilize in order to best serve the needs of each client. Be honest, but make certain to relay an account that reflects positively on you.

Familiarize yourself with the questions that an employer by law is not supposed to ask and prepare a response for the situation. For example, it is not appropriate for someone to ask if you have children or plan to have children in the near future. You can answer by saying "I can meet the work schedule this job requires."

Figure 23-6 contains examples of some common interview questions.

***Be Aware of Your Nonverbal Communication.*** Always start with a smile and a firm handshake. Those simple gestures convey your level of self-confidence and are indicators of how proficient your interpersonal skills may be. Relax, maintain good eye contact, and keep your posture controlled. Interviewers are aware that you may be nervous, but it should not be acutely obvious. Deliver your answers with a sense of energy. Organizations need employees who have a personable and enthusiastic presence.

- Tell me about yourself.

- Tell me about your relevant experience/clinical practicum.

- What did you like best about your clinical experiences?

- What was your worst clinical experience?

- What types of assessments/therapies do you feel comfortable administering?

- In what area do you think you need the most training/supervision?

- How would you implement an IEP?

- How would you keep track of client progress?

- How do you work with a patient who is making very little progress?

- How do you determine whether or not your service for a client is successful?

- What expectations do you have of your clients? Of their parents/family?

- How would you work with parents/family members of clients enrolled in your program?

- How would you relate your intervention to a client's classroom work?

- How would you handle a client who is openly frustrated and gives up?

- What types of professional conferences/workshops have you attended/are interested in attending?

- Would you feel comfortable presenting an in-service workshop to teachers, social workers, or nurses?

- Why did you choose speech–language pathology as a career?

- What do you find rewarding about this field?

- What do you consider to be your greatest strengths and weaknesses?

- What are your short-term and long-range career goals?

- What three characteristics describe you best?

- What are your three greatest accomplishments?

- Why should I hire you?

- How would you describe the ideal job for you?

*(continues)*

**Figure 23-6** Interview questions (*Sources*: American Speech–Language–Hearing Association, 2003; *Opportunities in Speech–Language Pathology Careers, 2002*)

- What qualities should a successful speech–language pathologist possess?

- What qualities should a good supervisor possess?

- What type of relationship would you like to establish with your supervisor?

- What kind of work environment/management style do you prefer?

- How has your education prepared you for a career in speech–language pathology?

- Describe your most rewarding academic experience.

- Why did you select your college or university?

- Do you think that your grades are a good indication of your ability level?

- How do you think you can make a meaningful contribution to our organization?

- Why do you want to work for this organization?

- What do you know about our organization?

- Describe a major problem you encountered and how you dealt with it.

- Describe a time when you failed to meet expectations on an assignment.

- Describe a time when someone criticized your work in front of others and your reaction to it.

- Describe a negative situation when it was important for you to maintain a positive attitude.

- Describe a time when you had to deal with a difficult person (client, classmate, co-worker, etc.).

- Describe a time when you got coworkers or classmates of dissimilar backgrounds, interests, or goals to collaborate productively on a project.

### Questions to Ask an Employer at an Interview

- What are some of the therapy objectives you would like accomplished?

**Figure 23-6** (*Continued*)

- What would my typical day entail?

- What qualities are you looking for in candidates for this position?

- What characteristics do successful employees of this organization seem to have in common?

- Do you encourage attendance at certain conferences, workshops, and other educational activities?

- How often are performance reviews given?

- How is one evaluated?

- What do you like best about your job? This organization?

- What are some of the more difficult challenges someone in this position tends to encounter?

- Who determines the size and composition of my caseload?

- What kind of equipment/instruments/resources do you have?

- Would you please describe typical client in this program?

- What is the next course of action? When should I expect to hear from you?

**Figure 23-6** (*Continued*)

***Speak in a Clear, Articulate, Specific Manner.*** This is not the time to be shy and reticent. At the same time, avoid rambling, discursive speeches. Take your time and think about your answers before communicating them. Recruiters are seeking resourceful, effective communicators who can summon up logical, rational responses to a wide variety of professional issues. Be able to succinctly show how you fit the position and the organization's climate. Give specific examples that demonstrate how your strengths fit the characteristics that are required of the position. Confidently assert the reasons you are a valuable asset to your chosen profession. Stay sincere, because it is very difficult to keep track of lies and even harder to live up to them on the job.

***Remain Positive.*** Show motivation and enthusiasm by explaining why you want the position. Be ready to identify the positive qualities you can bring to the organization. Avoid debasing a former employer or talking negatively about a past work experience. If you are asked to discuss a negative experience, relay how you turned it into a positive one and what you learned from it. Employers are looking for candidates who maintain a positive attitude and a team spirit even during adverse times.

***Refer to Sample Items.*** Consider bringing a portfolio containing samples of your project work, recommendation letters, thank-you letters received, awards, congratulatory letters, and/or performance evaluations. Refer to those samples when you are attempting to demonstrate something you mention. If you do use them, make certain you have copies of everything, in case an employer wants to hold on to some for review.

***Close Effectively.*** Closing effectively means ending the interview with well–thought out questions. Questions indicate interest and show that you have actually given the position much thought. Figure 23-6 also contains some examples of questions that you may consider asking the employer. Do not inquire about salary and benefits. Employers will divulge these details eventually, although maybe not until after they make an offer. Asking about salary conveys that you are more interested in the money than you are in the opportunity. Briefly summarize with some basic statements about how your aptitude and abilities fit in with the position. Ask what the next course of action is. Request business cards from your interviewers, and thank all for their time.

## After the Interview

***Send Thank-You Letters.*** Thank-you letters are not optional; they are essential and employers expect them. They should be mailed within 23 hours after the interview. You can type or e-mail your thank-you letter. Thank-you letters indicate that you are cordial and that you are grateful for the opportunity to interview. They also display your enthusiasm for the position you are seeking to attain. Thank all for the chance to interview, reminding them about the specific position for which you applied. The business cards you requested at the conclusion of each interview will be helpful when you are writing your thank-you letters. Reiterate your interest in the position and the organization, and mention the skills and qualities you can bring to the company that make you an ideal candidate for the position. Figure 23-7 is an example of a thank-you letter to an employer. The following suggestions can be used to create an effective thank-you letter.

- ***First Paragraph:*** Thank the interviewer for the opportunity to meet with them, stating the position for which you were interviewed and the date of the interview.

- ***Second Paragraph:*** Reemphasize how your skills and experiences might make you an ideal match for the position, mentioning something that is especially appealing.

- ***Third Paragraph:*** Reaffirm your interest in the position and the organization. State your willingness to provide additional information. Thank all interviewers for their time and consideration.

**Kerry J. Doe**
_____
123 State Road • Orland Park, Illinois 60462 • (708) 555-1111 • kdoe@mailbox.com

March 10, 2004

Melissa Smith
Assistant Superintendent
Fairview School District 123
7890 W. Main Street
Fairview, IL 61432

Dear Ms. Smith:

Thank you very much for interviewing me for the Speech Therapist-Clinical Fellowship position with your school district today. You and your colleagues provided me with a very warm reception and informative discussion.

My enthusiasm for working with your district was strengthened as a result of our meeting, and the opportunity is congruent with the type of experience I am seeking. As mentioned during our conversation, my experiences as a Speech Assistant and as a Student Clinician have prepared me extensively for the type of work required of a Speech Pathologist in a school environment. In addition, my positive interpersonal qualities, proficient analytical abilities, and strong communication skills would make me an ideal candidate for the position. Furthermore, my willingness to assist with your college mentoring program would enable me to be a versatile contributor to your organization.

Once again, I wish to reiterate my genuine interest in the position and your organization. If you have any questions, please contact me at (708) 555-1111. Thank you very much for your valuable time and consideration.

Sincerely,

*Kerry Doe*

Kerry Doe

**Figure 23-7** Thank-you letter *(Source: Delmar/Cengage Learning.)*

---

**Job Search Resources**

Not sure where to start your employment search? Try these resources:

- Directories of special education cooperatives/joint agreements
- Directories of public schools at http://www.ed.gov
- Directories of human care services
- ASHA Career Center/Placement Center at http://www.asha.org
- Job fairs (especially education and health care career fairs)
- College/university career center job listings
- Sunday newspaper classified advertisements
- Professional associations
- Networking
- Web pages

---

## CONCLUSION

Now that you have almost completed (or have completed) your course of study, it would be nice if there were a great job just waiting for you. Unfortunately, it is not quite as easy as that. Sometimes things work out such that a person gets the first job he or she applies for. Applying for jobs can often feel like a full-time job in itself, and it may take repeated interviews and a good amount of time before the right position is found. Be prepared to put in the time to first find jobs that are suited to your needs and interests, and then to create high-quality, error-free documents such as your résumé, cover letter, and thank-you letter. Close attention to detail with these steps is important to securing that job of your dreams. Although interviews are vital to prospective employers as they look for the right person for their position, interviews are your opportunity to decide whether a position, or employer, is the right fit for you. Just as the employer will screen out candidates who do not meet the organization's expectations or needs, you should screen out employers who do not fit your expectations and needs.

# PART 5

# Professional Associations

# The National Student Speech Language Hearing Association

## INTRODUCTION

The National Student Speech Language Hearing Association (NSSLHA) is a preprofessional membership association for students interested in the study of communication sciences and disorders (CSD). NSSLHA averages 12,000 members and has over 300 local chapters at colleges and universities throughout the United States, Canada, Greece, and Saudi Arabia. NSSLHA is a student-run association, independent of the professional association the American Speech–Language–Hearing Association (ASHA). The relationship between NSSLHA and ASHA is an advantage to students. Students who affiliate with NSSLHA at the undergraduate level and maintain membership throughout graduate study have greater access to academic resources, have more networking opportunities, and are better prepared for their professional careers. This chapter will provide an overview of the association and provide more details on the benefits of membership.

## WHY NATIONAL STUDENT SPEECH LANGUAGE HEARING ASSOCIATION?

Imagine being a member of a group of students that shares a similar interest, can provide resources that will benefit you as a student and as a professional, and allows you to have a leadership role in your future professional association. That group exists. A student looking for this type of access should join NSSLHA.

NSSLHA exists to provide students interested in CSD with a closer affiliation to professionals in the discipline. A student who chooses membership in NSSLHA is making an investment to become a better CSD professional. NSSLHA members learn, early in their careers, the value of advocacy, certification, continuing education, ethics, and research in contributing to their long-term success.

Any student, full-time or part-time, undergraduate or graduate, national or international, may apply for membership in NSSLHA. NSSLHA membership is not available to a student who has applied for or received the Certificate of Clinical Competence from ASHA.

Students can separately apply for membership to NSSLHA at the local and national levels. Moreover, students may affiliate with NSSLHA on the campus of their communication sciences program or apply directly to the national association for membership. However, they are strongly encouraged to apply to both. The national association offers benefits that are separate from what is available from the local chapter.

Figure 24-1 lists the top-10 benefits of membership in NSSLHA.

1. **Conversion Discount.** For every graduate student who has maintained 2 consecutive years of national student membership at the time of graduation, ASHA offers a discount off the initial dues and fees for ASHA membership and certification.

2. **Convention Discounts.** Every national student member who attends the annual ASHA convention (or other ASHA-sponsored professional event) receives a significant discount on the registration fee.

3. **Discounted Special Interest Division Membership.** ASHA Special Interest Divisions are groups of professionals and students who share an interest in one of 16 specialty areas (e.g., language, neurogenics, voice, hearing disorders). Members of NSSLHA can join a Special Interest Division for $10.

4. **NSSLHA Publications.** Members receive a subscription to the award-winning newsletter *NSSLHA Now!* and the highly regarded, peer-reviewed journal *Contemporary Issues in Communication Sciences and Disorders* (CICSD).

5. **ASHA Publications and HighWire.** In addition to receiving *The ASHA Leader*, members have access to all of ASHA's journals online, with unlimited searches of full-text articles through ASHA's HighWire site.

6. **In the Loop.** NSSLHA's monthly electronic newsletter keeps members updated on the latest programs, services, and events.

7. **Technical Assistance from ASHA.** NSSLHA members have unlimited access to all members-only content on the ASHA Web site, for unprecedented research and other resources for academic study.

8. **NSSLHA Online Community.** Members enjoy an online forum where they can exchange ideas and network with other audiology and speech–language pathology students.

9. **National Leadership Opportunities.** National student members are eligible to apply for positions on the executive council or serve on national committees and shape policies that impact students in communication sciences programs.

10. **Becoming a Better ASHA Member.** Without a doubt, the student who takes full advantage of national membership becomes a highly functioning ASHA member. Affiliating with the national association throughout academic study leads to a holistic ASHA professional who is knowledgeable advocate for the profession.

**Figure 24-1** Top 10 NSSLHA membership benefits *(Reprinted with permission by the National Student Speech Language Hearing Association NSSLHA Now! February 2007.)*

Joining the national association is easy:

- Join online through the NSSLHA Web site. Click on the "Join" link.
- Call the ASHA Action Center at 800-498-2071 and enroll over the telephone using a major credit card (MasterCard or Visa only).
- Ask the NSSLHA chapter at your university for an application and mail in your application with check, money order, or credit card information to NSSLHA, PO Box 1169, Rockville, MD 20850.

NSSLHA prepares students to be leaders in their future profession. What makes NSSLHA unique is that it is a national association governed by an executive council (EC) that consist of 11 NSSLHA members (students), who serve as regional councilors (RCs), and five ASHA members (faculty), who serve as consultants to the council.

Becoming a member of the council provides a student with an extraordinary leadership experience. Issues that affect students or the operation of the association are brought before the EC. The council is responsible for discussing those issues and determining a solution or a course of action in the best interest of the majority of the membership.

Students who have national membership in the association may apply for openings on the NSSLHA executive council. Applications and more information on the NSSLHA executive council are available on the NSSLHA Web site. Search for the "Council" link.

Figure 24-2 lists the advantages of applying for a position as an RC.

The executive council oversees the following programs and activities for students and local chapters:

- ***Advocacy Program for Students:*** A publication created by the council to teach students how to advocate for issues relevant to CSD and clients living with communication disorders.

- ***CICSD* Mentoring Program:** Could you use some support getting your research published? Any individual who has never published in a journal is eligible to participate in the *CICSD* Mentoring Program. Inclusion in this program does not guarantee acceptance and publication of your manuscript in *CICSD*. A $100 honorarium is awarded to student manuscripts accepted for publication.

- **Communication Science and Disorder Career Awareness:** Local chapters can register with the national office to receive complimentary and online materials to promote the professions to high school students, undergraduate students undecided about a major, and students enrolled in community colleges. Students are invited by the chapter to visit the CSD program to talk to professionals working in the field, tour a speech and hearing clinic, and to participate in a hearing screening.

- **Community Service Grants:** The NSSLHA executive council established a grant award program to fund local chapters that wish to provide resources to nonprofit organizations that assist others living with a communication disorder. NSSLHA chapters in good standing

1. **Easy Online Application.** Students may visit the "Council" page of the NSSLHA Web site to apply for a position online.

2. **Fun.** Students have an opportunity to work with other students and make long-lasting friendships.

3. **Savings.** Attend the ASHA convention and other activities and all your travel, lodging, and meals are covered by the national association.

4. **Advocacy.** Participate in Capitol Hill visits where you present current issues in communication sciences to your representatives in the House and Senate.

5. **Access.** Receive unrestricted access to individuals and resources that can positively influence your academic and professional development.

6. **National Exposure.** Have the opportunity to host sessions at state association conventions, facilitate presentations during NSSLHA Day, and represent the association at local and national events.

7. **Leadership Development.** Your council experience prepares you for leadership positions in state associations and ASHA.

8. **Participation.** You have voting responsibilities with the ASHA Audiology Council and Speech–Language–Pathology Council, the Board of Division Coordinators, and the Multicultural Issues Board.

9. **Influence.** You have direct influence over the programs, policies, and activities that affect members and the local chapters.

10. **Networking.** You enjoy direct access to other students and professional council members on a local, state, and national level.

**Figure 24-2.** Ten advantages of applying for a position as a regional councilor (*Source:* NSSLHA Now! *November 2008, pp. 6–7.)*

are eligible to receive matching funds assistance up to $1,000 to purchase equipment (e.g., augmentative and alternative communication [AAC] devices, computers, and/or peripheral computer devices) or other materials (e.g., clinical tests, software) to donate to a nonprofit organization.

- **McKinley Regional Project Grants:** NSSLHA chapters in good standing are eligible to receive grants up to $1,000 to support educational, clinical, and professional development activities for students in CSD programs. Regional Project Funds should be used to enable NSSLHA members to expand their knowledge of the profession through the development of materials, conferences, workshops, and sessions.

- **NSSLHA Day at the ASHA Convention:** The ASHA annual convention is a great opportunity for students and professionals to meet for discussions, workshops, and the presentation of papers and informal talks. In addition to the formal ASHA program, students can participate in NSSLHA-sponsored activities during the convention. These events are specifically for students and were developed by the student leaders serving on the NSSLHA executive council.

- **NSSLHA Honors Program:** The NSSLHA executive council annually recognizes individuals or NSSLHA chapters who make a significant contribution to furthering the association's mission. NSSLHA awards the Honors of NSSLHA, Chapter Advisor of the Year Honors, Chapter of the Year Honors, Member Honors, and the Editor's Award to promote the good work of students and professionals in the professions.

- **"NSSLHA Loves" Campaign:** Annually, the NSSLHA executive council selects a national organization working on behalf of individuals living with communication disorders and facilitates a fundraising campaign through the local chapters and national members.

  Since the inception of the "NSSLHA Loves" program in 1990, NSSLHA has raised over $220,000 in support of national organizations improving the quality of life for individuals with communication disorders.

- **NSSLHA Publications:** Members of the executive council are involved in the writing and publishing of *NSSLHA Now!* the associations newsletter; *Contemporary Issues in Communication Sciences and Disorders* (CICSD), the association's journal; and the *CSD Student Survival Guide* published by Delmar Cengage Learning.

## CONCLUSION

For any student, pursuing an academic career in communication sciences can be daunting. The key to getting through it is to align yourself with people and resources that will help you succeed. Joining NSSLHA is your first step.

# American Speech–Language–Hearing Association

## INTRODUCTION

Since its founding in 1925, American Speech–Language–Hearing Association (ASHA) remains one of the largest and most recognized organizations dedicated to the promotion of speech–language pathology and audiology. ASHA is the professional, scientific, and credentialing association for over 130,000 members and affiliates who are speech–language pathologists (SLPs), audiologists, and speech, language, and hearing scientists in the United States and internationally.

ASHA's mission is to empower and support SLPs, audiologists, and speech, language, and hearing scientists by:

- Advocating on behalf of persons with communication and related disorders
- Advancing communication science
- Promoting effective human communication

ASHA facilitates two separate functions for professional audiologists or SLPs: membership and certification. Membership and certification are mutually exclusive activities. A professional may become a member of ASHA without applying for certification, he or she may apply for certification without membership, or he or she may apply for both membership and certification. There are some advantages to having both. For instance, a certified member is able to provide clinical services and has access to ASHA technical assistance while working as a clinician.

ASHA provides graduate students who maintain 2 consecutive years of membership in the student association National Student Speech Language Hearing Association [NSSLHA] with a significant discount on the initial dues and fees of ASHA membership and certification. This provision is called the Conversion Discount. More information about the Conversion Discount is available on the ASHA Web site. Search for "Conversion Discount."

There are many other advantages to membership and certification in ASHA. This chapter will provide an overview of those benefits. This chapter will also discuss ASHA's primary networking and educational event, the ASHA convention. Attending the ASHA convention is one of the most valuable educational activities that students can partake in their preprofessional career. Figure 25-1 is a checklist for your first trip to the ASHA convention. These tips are followed by a primer on what to do once you are at the ASHA convention.

- [ ] Research Funding Opportunities for the Convention
- [ ] Volunteer at the ASHA Convention
- [ ] Organize a Fundraiser for Trip Expenses
- [ ] Register Early to Receive the "Early/Early Bird" Registration Fee
- [ ] Make Travel Arrangements for the Convention
- [ ] Find a Place to Stay
- [ ] Plan Your Commute to the Convention Center from Where You Stay
- [ ] Review the Convention Program Online and Set Up a Flexible Schedule
- [ ] Get Handy with Handouts
- [ ] Bring Your Convention Registration Materials to the Convention
- [ ] Bring a Good Pair of Walking Shoes, Professional Clothing, and Business Cards
- [ ] Attend Preconference Workshops
- [ ] Visit the NSSLHA Booth
- [ ] Explore the Exhibit Hall
- [ ] Visit the ASHA Service Center
- [ ] Attend the Poster Sessions
- [ ] Participate in the NSSLHA Day Events
- [ ] Attend the Graduate School Fair
- [ ] Attend the Career Fair with Your Résumé Even if You are Not Currently Looking for a Job
- [ ] Attend the NSSLHA Executive Council Meeting
- [ ] Join your Colleagues at Special Events
- [ ] Meet and Greet
- [ ] Bring Extra Money

**Figure 25-1** Checklist for your first trip to the ASHA convention *(Source: Delmar/ Cengage Learning.)*

## ASHA MEMBERSHIP

Membership in ASHA provides all the resources and information you need to be successful at your job, advance your career, and serve your profession. The minimum requirement for ASHA membership is a graduate degree or its equivalent with major emphasis in audiology; speech–language pathology; or speech, language, or hearing science.

ASHA members receive the following:

- **Cutting-Edge Professional Publications.** Members have free online access to the full text of all four ASHA journals—American Journal of Audiology; American Journal of Speech–Language Pathology; Journal of Speech, Language, and Hearing Research; and Language, Speech, and Hearing Services in School.

- **Continuing Education Opportunities.** Members earn continuing educational units (CEUs), which are required to keep licensure up to date, for activities such as presenting at conferences, authoring and publishing journal articles, earning academic credit, participating in journal study groups, or learning related to clinical fellow supervision.

- **Complete, Unrestricted Access to ASHA's Web Site.** Members have unlimited access to the award-winning Web site, the largest, most comprehensive resource for audiologists and SLPs online today.

- **Annual Convention.** Members attend the ASHA convention at a discounted rate. The ASHA convention is the largest gathering of speech, language, and hearing professionals in the world. Read more about the ASHA convention in this chapter.

- **Technical Assistance.** ASHA staff can help practicing SLPs and audiologists get information about planning, funding strategies, identifying appropriate agencies and agency representatives, and developing proposal concepts.

- **Special Interest Divisions.** Thousands of ASHA members are staying on the cutting-edge of issues and concerns within their areas of interest through membership in one or more of ASHA's Special Interest Divisions. More information about the Divisions is available in Chapter 26.

- **Discounts on ASHA Products and Services.** Members receive discounts from 20% to 50% off nonmember prices for reference books and handbooks, continuing education (CE) products, multicultural resources, specialty products to promote your services to colleagues and consumers, and much more.

Additional benefits for ASHA members are the following:

- Professional liability and auto/home insurance programs
- Subaru–VIP Partners Program
- Avis Auto Rental
- Bank of America MasterCard and Visa

ASHA members are bound by ASHA's Code of Ethics. The Code of Ethics is rules and principles that guide the professional conduct of audiologists and SLPs. More detailed information about ASHA's Code of Ethics is available on the ASHA Web site. Search for "Code of Conduct."

# ASHA CERTIFICATION

Holding ASHA certification means holding the nationally recognized credential, the Certificate of Clinical Competence (CCC), a professional certification that represents a level of excellence in audiology (CCC-A) or speech–language pathology (CCC-SLP). Holding ASHA certification offers increased opportunities for employment, mobility, career advancement, professional credibility, and more, because it is recognized by nearly every state's regulatory agency. The CCC validates and provides assurance to consumers and clients; other health care professionals; and employers, state licensure boards, and third-party payers that through participation in continuous professional development activities they can be confident certificate holders are keeping up with rapid changes in the professions' scopes of practice. The CCCs are a basic requirement to practice audiology or speech–language pathology.

More information on the CCCs is available in this guide and can be found on the ASHA Web site. Search for "Certification."

# THE ASHA CONVENTION

The ASHA convention is an inspiring experience that all communication sciences and disorders (CSD) students should participate in at least once. Over 10,000 students; audiologists; SLPs; and speech, language, and hearing scientists; parents, and related professionals attend the annual convention each November. When you walk into the spacious convention building, you will probably feel a bit overwhelmed. There is so much to see and do that you might miss out if you do not know what to look for. If you have never been to a convention, you probably have questions about what it is like. Figure 25-1 is a checklist to help you prepare for your first ASHA convention. Following those tips is one of the suggestions on how to get the most out of the ASHA convention experience as a student.

## Research Funding Opportunities for the Convention

There are several resources available to help students defray their costs to attend the ASHA convention. NSSLHA hosts an Ambassador's contest among the local NSSLHA chapters. Chapters selected to serve as Ambassador's during NSSLHA Day may receive up to $1,000 for their participation. Information and an application for the NSSLHA Day Ambassador's Program is available on the Chapters page of the NSSLHA Web site.

ASHA makes travel grants available to students who are presenting their research during the ASHA convention. A search of the ASHA Web site for ASHA Award Programs will provide links to several student research grants and other convention-related opportunities.

Also, some campuses have funds set aside for students to attend educational events. As you might imagine, these funds are not usually advertised. Contact your campus's student organization board to see if you and/or your NSSLHA chapter qualify. Resources may also be available through the national association.

## Volunteer at the ASHA Convention

Students are eligible to apply for volunteer opportunities during the ASHA convention. Students selected by ASHA to volunteer will receive a refund equivalent to the cost of the early-bird registration fee. The application for volunteers is available on the Convention page of the ASHA Web site. To be chosen as a volunteer, you need to fill out a volunteer application form in May or June. Make sure you have renewed your membership in NSSLHA because preferences are given to its members.

A volunteer's role at convention is to meet and greet convention goers, provide directions, and assist with crowd control at registration, events, or sessions. ASHA will require your assistance for at least 8 hours. That might seem like a long time, but you will be busy the entire time. You will still be able to participate in convention activities. Most of the time you will be allowed to work at or near sessions/events that you want to attend.

## Organize a Fundraiser for Trip Expenses

Often, local NSSLHA chapters hold fundraisers to help cover the costs of attending the ASHA Convention. If yours does not, ask if you can set up fundraising activities, such as bake sales, cookbooks, products with your school's logo on them. Also, some campuses have funds set aside for students to attend educational events. As you might imagine, these funds are not usually advertised. Contact your campus' student organization board to see if you and/or your NSSLHA chapter qualify. Resources may also be available through the national association.

## Register Early to Receive the "Early/Early Bird" Registration Fee

The cost of convention varies from year to year, but members of NSSLHA receive a significant discount to attend the ASHA convention.

## Make Travel Arrangements for the Convention

Traditionally, the convention is the week before Thanksgiving, from Thursday until Saturday. This period can be a hectic time for many students, and depending on what your travel plans may be for Thanksgiving, if you want to attend ASHA convention as well, you should start planning well in advance. The ASHA Web site has information on the cost, location, and dates of the convention each year. If you look early enough, you might be able to find an affordable flight. Try travel search engines. However, driving may be cheaper if you can carpool with others and split the cost of gas and parking.

Do a search using an online map service to see how far the convention is from your front door. If you opt to drive, call your hotel to see if you have to pay extra for parking. If you plan to fly, you should see if your hotel has complimentary transportation services to and from the airport or train station.

## Find a Place to Stay

If you do not have any friends or relatives to stay with near the convention city, make reservations at a hotel or student hostel. Most students find roommates from their university program and split the cost of a hotel room. ASHA has lists of hotels in the convention city on their Web site. These hotels may have a reduced rate for ASHA convention attendees and have shuttles to and from the convention center. Some students stay at student hostels, which are found in most major cities. Hostels are places designated specifically for students, where they can stay for a relatively inexpensive rate. They do not come with the amenities of the average hotel, but the prices are much lower. Check the ASHA Web site to identify the student hostel in the city of the next ASHA convention.

## Plan Your Commute to the Convention Center from Where You Stay

Although there may be ASHA-provided shuttles to and from some hotels, they may not be available where you are staying. Therefore, expect to take public transportation, such as a bus, train, or subway. Walking is always an option if you are within a few miles of the convention center. Your hotel or the hostel can assist you in finding the best way to get to the convention center.

## Review the Convention Program Online and Set Up a Flexible Schedule

Planning ahead of time will keep you focused on presentations that initially piqued your interest. Use ASHA's online Scheduler/Itinerary Planner to browse more than 1,400 education sessions and conference events. During the ASHA sessions, speakers usually discuss their cutting-edge research. Some sessions are at the introductory level and others are at the advanced level. If a topic interests you or corresponds to a research project you are working on, be sure to arrive early to get a good seat.

## Get Handy with Handouts

Handouts for many sessions are available through ASHA's Online Scheduler. Search for the Annual Convention on the ASHA Web site for a link to the convention handouts.

# Bring Your Convention Registration Materials to the Convention

If you register early, ASHA will mail you a badge and tickets for any prereg-istered events (e.g., NSSLHA Luncheon and Awards Ceremony). Make sure to bring these materials along with you to the convention. Your badge and tickets are required for entry into all events. If you do forget them, these items can be reissued at the Convention registration area, but be prepared to wait in a line.

# Bring a Good Pair of Walking Shoes, Professional Clothing, and Business Cards

If you have never attended a convention or event at a major convention center before, you will most likely be amazed at how huge these buildings are. Once you are in the convention center, you will be doing a lot of walking between sessions, events, and the exhibitor hall where products and services are featured. Plus, you will most likely be walking to and from your hotel or to other points of interest in the city. Good walking shoes are a must! You will be interacting with many professionals, some of whom are highly respected and influential in the field, and you will want to present yourself as a professional as well. You should wear professional clothing that is comfortable (e.g., women can wear dress pants and a blouse or business skirt set; men can wear dress pants, shirt, and tie and dress jacket if preferred). Although jeans and casual clothing are not prohibited, this convention is a professional event, and you should show respect to your colleagues by dressing appropriately. Also, bring business cards, which are helpful because you will do a lot of networking. You will interact with professionals and students who you may want to keep in contact with after the convention. Purchase business card paper from an office supply store and use a word-processing program such as Microsoft Word to format your own cards in order to easily handout your contact information.

# Attend Preconference Workshops

ASHA Special Interest Division usually sponsors workshops a day or two before the convention begins. During these workshops, speakers often present papers on a disorder and how to treat it; however, the topics may vary. Generally, you are required to preregister for workshops and pay extra. Moreover, if you are a member of the ASHA Special Interest Division that hosts the workshop, you may receive a significant discount.

# Visit the NSSLHA Booth

The NSSLHA booth is a great starting point for the ASHA convention. You can pick up the NSSLHA convention brochure and ask any questions about the convention, NSSLHA membership, or academic issues. While at the NSSLHA booth, pick up a ribbon to attach to your nametag that identifies you are an NSSLHA member or a local chapter president.

## Explore the Exhibit Hall

The exhibit hall is filled with companies and services displaying and selling their most up-to-date products. You will find publishers selling books and software, usually at a significant discount. In fact, if you know that you need a particular book for an upcoming class, you may want to take advantage of the special convention discount. You can also pick up a lot of freebies at this event, such as tote bags, pens, highlighters, key chains, penlights (which are especially useful for oral mechanism examinations), and notepads. However, choose wisely when taking items. Otherwise, you will end up with a lot of unnecessary junk to pack on your way back. The exhibit hall is usually open on Thursday, Friday, and Saturday of convention.

## Visit the ASHA Service Center

The ASHA service center, located in the center of the exhibit hall, is a smaller version of the national office. Students may go there to update their contact information, to learn about their Conversion status, to talk with a certification case manager, or to get information about ASHA membership.

## Attend the Poster Sessions

Providing excellent forums for one-on-one discussion of recent research, poster sessions let you see a great deal in a short amount of time. In poster presentations, investigators summarize their research on a poster and give you a brief explanation. Many poster presentations are given in a gigantic room. Attendees can walk up and down the rows of posters and stop to read the posters that interest them. Usually someone from the research team is present to explain the poster. Presentations change throughout the day, so it is helpful to identify when the posters that interest you will be available by looking on the ASHA Web site.

## Participate in the NSSLHA Day Events

Take advantage of a day of programming aimed at students and student issues. The day begins with professional development series that tackle preprofessional matters that are important to students. You may find sessions about the Praxis Series examination and information about clinical fellowships, *how to select* a job setting, *how to prepare* a résumé, and *how to select* a graduate school. The professional development series is then followed by the NSSLHA Luncheon and Award Ceremony, where local chapters and individuals on both the national and the local level are recognized for their contributions to NSSLHA. The day ends with a fun activity, The Battle of the Regions: NSSLHA Knowledge Bowl. The knowledge bowl presents Praxis-like questions in a jeopardy-style battle. One team per region is picked. The winning team is eligible for cash awards up to $1,000. The full schedule of NSSLHA Day activities is available on the NSSLHA Day page of the NSSLHA Web site.

## Attend the Graduate School Fair

NSSLHA in partnership with ASHA sponsors the Graduate School Fair (GSF). The GSF provides students the opportunity to meet with representatives from communication sciences programs nationally and internationally in one convenient location. Traditionally, the GSF is held the Thursday and Friday of Convention from noon to 4:00 pm. The programs that exhibit on Thursday are doctoral focused. The programs that exhibit on Friday are focused on recruiting students into masters-level programs.

## Attend the Career Fair with Your Résumé Even if You are Not Currently Looking for a Job

Meet with an employer participating in the Résumé Star Program for a 15-minute session and get tips on polishing your résumé for college applications, scholarships, internships, or simply to land your first job. You must arrive at the career fair with at least a draft of a résumé. You may have the opportunity to have a future employer edit your résumé. The résumé review is on a first-come-first-served basis, so you may have to wait in line until someone is able to help you. Also, this is a great time to look for and apply for jobs. Stop by the Career Fair registration desk for a list of participating employers, or look for the Résumé Star logo on employers' booths.

## Attend the NSSLHA Executive Council Meeting

The NSSLHA executive council holds one of its general business meetings during the ASHA convention. These meetings are open for NSSLHA members where they can share their ideas. Members interested in attending these meeting should contact their Regional Councilor or the national office for meeting times and locations.

## Join your Colleagues at Special Events

Join hundreds of ASHA professionals and NSSLHA members during events such as the Opening General Session, the ASHA Awards ceremony, or the NSSLHA Luncheon and Awards Ceremony. Hear a keynote address from some of the disciplines' most noted professionals. Get motivated about your profession through words of encouragement by your elected leaders. Celebrate your colleagues' academic and professional accomplishments.

## Meet and Greet

Seek out professionals and researchers whose work you have read in textbooks and journal articles. Introduce yourself and express your appreciation for their contribution to our discipline.

## Bring Extra Money

Accidents and unexpected events can happen. If you are driving, your car could break down and you will need to pay for repairs. If you are flying, your flight might be delayed or canceled, and you may need to buy food. Be prepared so you are not stranded anywhere.

## CONCLUSION

The ASHA convention has much to offer students and professionals in CSD. You can learn about the most cutting-edge research, attend sessions pertaining to your particular areas of interest, access a wide range of products and services in the exhibit hall, find out more about potential graduate schools and job opportunities, and, of course, meet CSD students from around the country for some fun social events. It is everything related to speech, language, hearing, and swallowing, all in one place, at one time. Attending the convention as a student is excellent preparation for attending it later as a certified practicing professional.

# CHAPTER 26

# Special Interest Divisions

## INTRODUCTION

Members of the American Speech–Language–Hearing Association (ASHA) join one of ASHA's 16 Special Interest Divisions (generally referred to as the *Divisions*) to exchange professional and scientific information with other members with similar professional interests. Each Special Interest Division is a community solely focused on a professional area of practice or work setting. National Student Speech Language Hearing Association (NSSLHA) members pay $10 to join a Division, whereas ASHA members pay $35 to join a Division. Students with membership in a Division have access to all the same benefits as those of members of ASHA who join a Division but are unable to vote or hold office. Some of the benefits for Division members are access to *Perspectives* publications (which offer continuing education self-studies), ASHA Pre-Convention Workshops and ASHA Convention Short Courses, grant competitions, Web forums, and e-mail lists that enable affiliates to ask questions that will be answered by some of the leading professionals within that specific interest. To learn more about the specific benefits of each Division, search for "Divisions" on the ASHA Web site.

The current list of ASHA's 16 Special Interest Divisions is as follows:

1. Language Learning and Education
2. Neurophysiology and Neurogenic Speech and Language Disorders
3. Voice and Voice Disorders
4. Fluency and Fluency Disorders
5. Speech Science and Orofacial Disorders
6. Hearing and Hearing disorders: Research and Diagnostics
7. Aural Rehabilitation and Its Instrumentation
8. Hearing Conservation and Occupational Audiology
9. Hearing and Hearing Disorders in Childhood
10. Issues in Higher Education
11. Administration and Supervision
12. Augmentative and Alternative Communication
13. Swallowing and Swallowing Disorders (Dysphagia)

14. Communication Disorders and Sciences in Culturally and Linguistically Diverse (CLD) Populations

15. Gerontology

16. School-Based Issues

In this chapter, representatives from all Divisions share why they are interested in their specific specialty area, what their specific area involves, and advice for students pursuing a communication sciences and disorders (CSD) career in each of these Special Interest Divisions. More information about the Divisions is available on the ASHA Web site. Search for "Special Interest Divisions."

# DIVISION 1—LANGUAGE LEARNING AND EDUCATION

Responses by Lynne E. Hewitt, Ph.D., 2008–2010

**Q. *How did you become interested in this subject area?***

**A.** I became interested in working in schools initially because I love children and I love advocating for children. I enjoy the dynamic environment of the schools; you definitely do not do the same thing every day. You will learn something new every day. Schools provide opportunity to be a part of both educational and health related issues. There is a multitude of opportunities to collaborate with other professionals. The work hours and school vacations are great. Also, being part of the largest segment of ASHA members, over 50% of ASHA members have chosen to work in schools, provides an extensive supportive network.

**Q. *What does this subject area involve?***

**A.** Child language development and disorders is a broad area, and like the rest of speech–language pathology, it has an expanding scope of practice. Skilled practitioners working with children who have developmental language impairments need to have a sophisticated grasp of language on many levels. In modern practice, some understanding of the diversity of human languages is critical. Children on your caseloads may speak or have family members who speak a wide array of the world's languages. Practitioners in child language base their clinical decision-making on their knowledge of typical language development, so it is crucial to understand the development of child language. In order to adequately serve this population, you will also need to have extensive knowledge about cognitive, emotional, sensory, and neurological aspects of development. Speech–language pathologists (SLPs) working with children with language disorders use a great deal of standardized test instruments, so knowledge of contemporary test construction is needed in order to select and interpret formal tests. Assessment is more than just formal tests. We use our knowledge of language to informally assess a child's overall language development by analyzing language samples, and we work with caregivers and teachers to better understand a child's strengths and weaknesses at home and school. Finally, all SLPs are ethically bound to use the best available evidence to support their practice, so a good grasp of the intervention research is very important.

**Q. What do students need to know if they want to pursue an education and/or career in this subject area?**

**A.** Practitioners in child language development and disorders have the opportunity to work in many settings, including both inpatient and outpatient medical facilities, private practice, birth-to-three agencies, as well as private and public schools. The schools are the largest employers of SLPs, and one of the largest portions of a schools-based caseload is disorders impacting language development. A pediatric language caseload will include children affected by a range of disorders, so familiarity with special characteristics of developmental disorders is important. Some individuals choose to pursue specialized training in autism or learning disabilities, and all practitioners working with pediatric language will need some familiarity with these and other developmental disorders. When working with this particular population, one role of the SLP is to promote and support the development of literacy because research reveals there is a link between language and reading. SLPs working with children will also be working with families, so training in counseling and family-centered practice is vital. If you are interested in child language as a career focus, it is a great idea to take a foreign language while in college and pursue electives in linguistics, psycholinguistics, and literacy.

# DIVISION 2—NEUROPHYSIOLOGY AND NEUROGENIC SPEECH AND LANGUAGE DISORDERS

Responses by Janet P. Patterson, 2006–2008, Coordinator

**Q. How did you become interested in this subject area?**

**A.** I became interested in this profession after shadowing a speech–language pathologist. The array of courses offered in the major was attractive, particularly the anatomy courses and neurology courses. The idea of applying information to treatment and helping people resonated with me. As I progressed through the major, I became increasingly interested in neurology, the brain–behavior relationship, and communication disorders following brain injuries.

**Q. What does this subject area involve?**

**A.** This subject area, neurogenic communication disorders, involves understanding neurology; the brain–behavior relationship; symptoms of various disorders such as aphasia and apraxia of speech; diseases such as Parkinson's disease or amyotrophic lateral sclerosis; clinical practice research; evidence-based practice; and learning theory. Moreover, it involves determining an individual's diagnosis and presenting symptoms, considering the individual's psychosocial status and family support system, evaluating the individual's functional communication ability, and planning treatment for the communication disorder as the individual learns to live with the neurogenic communication disorder.

**Q. *What do students need to know if they want to pursue an education and/or career in this subject area?***

**A.** As with any area of speech–language pathology, in order to practice, an individual must hold the Certificate of Clinical Competence from ASHA, which entails completing a master's degree. In addition, specialty recognition from the Academy of Neurologic Communication Disorders & Sciences further confirms an individual's expertise in treating children or adults with neurogenic communication disorders.

Part of the preprofessional and continuing education in this area is coursework in aphasia, motor speech disorders, dementia, cognitive–communication disorders, traumatic brain injury, and neurology. In addition, coursework in psycholinguistics, neurolinguistics, cognitive psychology, neuropsychology, statistics, and learning theory contributes to an understanding of the assessment and treatment of clients with neurogenic communication disorders.

A clinician working in a medical setting with clients who have neurogenic communication disorders must be able to work with a team of medical and rehabilitation professionals and understand information relevant to the practice setting, such as medical terminology, medications, patient effects on communication, and medical coding systems. Treatment for neurogenic communication disorders can be delivered in individual or group sessions. Clinicians must understand the principles of therapy in these settings and how to facilitate communication for clients who have communication deficits. Many clients who have neurogenic communication disorders will not recover completely, but they do have the potential to develop functional communication skills.

# DIVISION 3—VOICE AND VOICE DISORDERS

Responses by Brian E. Petty, 2008–2010, Steering Committee Member

**Q. *How did you become interested in this subject area?***

**A.** I was an opera singer before I was a speech pathologist. During my master's degree in the school of music at Ohio State, I was required to take a number of courses in a field related to vocal music. I chose Mike Trudeau's voice disorders class in communication disorders, and I enjoyed it immensely. After graduating and working for a while, I chose to return to school to complete a second master's degree in speech/hearing science.

**Q.** *What does this subject area involve?*

**A.** This subject area, voice and swallowing disorders, involves the diagnosis and treatment of voice, resonance, and swallowing disorders.

**Q.** *What do students need to know if they want to pursue an education and/or career in this subject area?*

**A.** Choose a graduate program that offers specific concentration in voice and swallowing. I would recommend choosing a program affiliated with a medical school or that runs a clinic specific to voice disorders. Work with your adviser to get as much instruction in voice as you can. Go to voice meetings and ASHA. Talk with people on Division 3's Listserve and ask for some recommendations. Most of all, I would recommend starting out as a generalist, as clinical fellowships in voice are hard to come by. A little professional flexibility will also make you more marketable.

# DIVISION 4—FLUENCY AND FLUENCY DISORDERS

• • • • • • • • • • • • • •

Responses by Vivian Sisskin, 2006–2008, Coordinator

**Q.** *How did you become interested in this subject area?*

**A.** As an undergraduate studying psychology at UCLA, I took a course in the psychology of communication disorders taught by Joseph Sheehan. Dr. Sheehan was a person who stuttered himself and directed a clinic on campus providing group therapy for the treatment of stuttering. He was a powerful instructor. His theories demonstrated the paradoxical nature of stuttering, for example, that people who stutter often stutter more when they are trying to hide it. I was fascinated with the complexities of stuttering, how many people who stutter could be completely covert (hide it successfully), and how speaking fears and resulting avoidance behavior could impact all facets of a person's life. I observed at the clinic, volunteered my time, and soon Dr. Sheehan became my teacher and mentor. I knew then that I wanted to learn all I could about fluency disorders. My goal was to specialize in treating stuttering.

**Q.** *What does this subject area involve?*

**A.** There are many types of fluency disorders. Persistent developmental stuttering is just one. Disfluent speech can also result from neurological disorders, psychological conditions, and linguistic weakness. In addition to learning about normal and disordered speech fluency, specialists in this

area will need to learn about language development and brain functioning. Learning theory is also important because many of the symptoms
of stuttering result from the person's effort to cope with the frustration
and embarrassment associated with disfluent speech. Counseling skills
are essential during the course of treatment and in helping parents and
teachers understand ways they can help their children and students who
stutter.

**Q. What do students need to know if they want to pursue
an education and/or career in this subject area?**

**A.** Students will find that there is a great demand in the workplace for clinicians and researchers who specialize in fluency disorders. Many clinicians feel insecure about their skills in working with people who have
fluency disorders, perhaps due to limited training and experience. Opportunities are plentiful for those who pursue education or a career in
this area. We do not know the cause of stuttering, and there are exciting
ongoing research projects to increase our understanding of the role of
genetics in stuttering, the motor and linguistic skills of those who stutter, and the various factors that might influence unaided recovery from
stuttering in young children. We still have a lot to learn about the kinds
of treatment programs that lead to lasting improvements in both speech
fluency and attitudes/emotions that impact communication. Furthermore,
we are only beginning to explore how prescription drugs and electronic
devices might be used in the comprehensive treatment of stuttering.
There are so many avenues of interest to explore!

# DIVISION 5—SPEECH SCIENCE AND OROFACIAL DISORDERS

• • • • • • • • • • • • • •

Responses by Mary O'Gara, 2007–2009, Associate Coordinator

**Q. How did you become interested in this subject area?**

**A.** I was exposed to this area of speech pathology as a teacher prior to
admission to graduate school. My graduate professors at Northwestern
University (Dr. Roger Dalston, Dr. Judith Trost-Cardamone, and Dr. Jeri
Logemann) fueled my passion for working with this population. I love
working with this fascinating group of clients with clefts and other craniofacial differences and the passionate professionals who engage in team
care. It is such a privilege to witness the growth and development of
babies who become communicatively competent children and later go
on to become productive adults.

**Q. What does this subject area involve?**

**A.** In a nutshell, caring for children with clefts and other craniomaxillofacial
differences involves (1) knowledge of the anatomy, physiology, and neurology of the vocal tract; (2) knowledge of the impact that velopharyngeal

dysfunction has on phonological development, resonance airflow control, and, sometimes, laryngeal function; (3) the ability to work within the context of a multidisciplinary team to achieve a coordinated treatment plan; and (4) willingness to engage long-term relationships with clients in a family-centered environment.

**Q.** *What do students need to know if they want to pursue an education and/or career in this subject area?*

**A.** You are needed and valued in this fascinating area of speech and language pathology. Choose a mentor, engage in learning the necessary skills, join Division 5, and enjoy a productive career in cleft/craniofacial care!

## DIVISION 6—HEARING AND HEARING DISORDERS: RESEARCH AND DIAGNOSTIC

Responses by Jennifer J. Lister, 2008–2010, Steering Committee Member

**Q.** *How did you become interested in this subject area?*

**A.** As a high school student, I had a great interest in helping people and a slightly greater interest in technology. I realized that my weak stomach (blood makes me extremely nauseous) precluded a career in medicine or nursing, so I started college with a major in computer science. At the end of my junior year, I was doing well in computer science, but realized that I was not passionate about the topic and felt detached from people. I still wanted to "help people," but I had no idea how to go about doing this. A friend was majoring in speech–language pathology and was clearly passionate about the field. Intrigued, I took a survey course in communication sciences and disorders. It included modules on speech and hearing science, phonetics, voice, fluency, language development/disorders, and other major topics in the field. I loved it! Here was a field in which I could help people, but it did not involve (much) blood and gore. Great! Technology played a big part too. Even better! I changed majors. After taking (and comparing) a course in language development and a course in hearing science, I realized that the field of audiology was more to my liking than speech–language pathology. I loved all the tests and instruments in audiology and the emphasis on diagnostics instead of long-term therapy. I wanted to help people immediately, after an hour or so of testing, not after months and months of therapy. I found something I was passionate about, and the more I learned about audiology, the more I loved it.

**Q.** *What does this subject area involve?*

**A.** Audiology involves problem solving, conducting tests, and using many different instruments to diagnose a hearing or balance disorder.

Audiology involves technology, fitting hearing aids and other listening devices to specific patients and specific hearing losses so that the patient may maximize his or her use of sound. Also, it involves counseling, helping people understand and cope with their hearing loss. Every patient is different and presents a different problem to solve, and hearing aid technology changes very quickly. So, audiologists are rarely bored; there is always a new challenge to tackle.

**Q. *What do students need to know if they want to pursue an education and/or career in this subject area?***

**A.** To become an audiologist, you must be ready to pursue a 4-year undergraduate degree followed by a 4-year doctoral degree. The topic of the undergraduate degree is not critical; many audiology doctoral programs accept students with undergraduate degrees in psychology, premedicine, engineering, biology, and business (just to name a few). An undergraduate degree in communication sciences and disorders will prepare you well for pursuit of a doctoral degree in audiology, however. The 4-year doctoral degree program in audiology is quite rigorous and includes practical clinical experiences as well as traditional didactic courses. Careers in audiology are varied and you may work in a medical, industrial, or educational setting.

# DIVISION 7—AURAL REHABILITATION AND ITS INSTRUMENTATION

Responses by Joseph J. Montano, 2005–2007, Coordinator

**Q. *How did you become interested in this subject area?***

**A.** I began to develop an interest in aural rehabilitation during my clinical fellowship. I was employed as an audiologist in a sheltered adult workshop for individuals with developmental disabilities. Many of my clients with Down syndrome had minimal hearing loss, and I wanted to provide them with some kind of treatment. I decided to establish a "listening group." Auditory training exercises and communication strategies were the initial activities. I quickly learned, when given the opportunity, people can be very self-expressive. What started out as a simple listening group grew into my first experience with audiologic counseling. Since that time, I've incorporated aural rehabilitation into all my work settings, including hospital, university, and long-term care.

**Q. *What does this subject area involve?***

**A.** Audiologic rehabilitation is the foundation of audiology. Our profession developed largely out of the aural rehabilitation programs established through the military during World War II. Even though the primary emphasis of audiology has shifted from rehabilitation to diagnostics, most people still consider diagnostics an integral component of aural rehabilitation. Basically, the goal of aural rehabilitation is to reduce or avoid the limitations that hearing loss can impose on communication and function. While there are many formal tests and assessment measures used, helping a person adjust to the loss of hearing is crucial. With this in mind, counseling is the heart and soul of aural rehabilitation, and amplification, auditory, speechreading, and communication training are tools available to the audiologist to enable self-adjustment to hearing loss.

**Q.** *What do students need to know if they want to pursue an education and/or career in this subject area?*

**A.** Students need to understand the impact of hearing loss on clients' ability to function within their environments and with their communication partners. In order for that understanding to occur, students need to be aware of the implications of how hearing loss goes beyond the audiogram. The audiogram is limited to the nature and degree of the hearing loss, but it does not tell us any information about its impact on a client's real-life functioning. Courses need to focus on the rehabilitative aspects of our professions and should not limit knowledge to diagnostics. Counseling needs to be infused in all coursework, and self-assessment needs to become as routine as speech audiometry in the diagnostic arsenal. Aural rehabilitation is one of our professional purposes, so it should be a significant component of our career regardless of employment setting.

# DIVISION 8—HEARING CONSERVATION AND OCCUPATIONAL AUDIOLOGY

Responses by Marjorie A. M. Grantham, 2008–2010, Steering Committee Member

**Q.** *How did you become interested in this subject area?*

**A.** I was a premedicine student at The University of Texas at Austin, when I took a course in communication sciences and disorders. I really enjoyed the subject, so I spoke with Dr. Fred Martin about the wisdom of changing from premedicine to audiology. He advised me, I changed my major, and I have never regretted this decision for a moment. As an Army Medic while I was studying at The University of Texas, I had the opportunity to test hearing and educate soldiers regarding preserving their hearing when I was conducting physical exams. I really liked the Army Hearing Conservation Program model, and this started me on my way to 16 years of working in hearing loss prevention.

**Q.** *What does this subject area involve?*

**A.** This field, hearing conservation and occupational audiology, requires that we use evidence-based practice to provide our patients with the very best hearing protectors, communications systems, and hearing loss prevention education. Moreover, it requires ongoing professional development and maintaining constant communication with experts in hearing conservation across disciplines.

**Q.** *What do students need to know if they want to pursue an education and/or career in this subject area?*

**A.** Take a Council for Accreditation in Occupational Hearing Conservation (CAOHC) course. CAOHC is the recognized national leader in training and certification in hearing loss prevention. Join the National Hearing Conservation Association (NHCA) and attend their conferences. NHCA is the national leader in bringing the hearing loss prevention experts together, and their conferences are spectacular for the cutting-edge information and quality presentations they provide.

## DIVISION 9—HEARING AND HEARING DISORDERS IN CHILDHOOD

Responses by Gayla Hutsell Guignard, 2008–2010, Coordinator

**Q.** *How did you become interested in this subject area?*

**A.** I became interested in childhood hearing and hearing disorders (specifically audiology and aural habilitation) toward the end of undergraduate school. I specifically became interested in children after I arrived at graduate school and had a clinical practicum experience at The University of Tennessee Child Hearing Services. I was amazed when I saw and heard children with severe-to-profound and profound hearing losses listening, talking, and thriving in life! I knew right away that working with kids who had no speech and language skills and helping them achieve communicative competence through spoken language therapy and a successful experience in mainstream education was for me. I've never known another group of children with more potential for improved outcomes than this group of children, and I've really enjoyed working with their dedicated parents over the years as well.

**Q.** *What does this subject area involve?*

**A.** The specialty area of aural habilitation involves knowledge and skills in both audiology and speech–language pathology. Additional knowledge in deaf education is a bonus, but not necessarily required. Find an audiologist or speech–language pathologist, with specialized training and skills in aural habilitation, who can mentor you as you develop clinical skills. You will also need to learn as much as you can about developmental milestones, hearing disorders, genetics, bilingual education, and children with additional exceptionalities, educational laws, and how they apply to children with special needs, and how to work with children within the family context. A strong desire to work closely with individual children, parents, and teams of professionals is highly important. If you are a loner and do not enjoy people, this is probably not an area of the field in which you might want to develop expertise.

The specialty area of pediatric audiology involves knowledge and skills in screening, assessment, and follow-up of very young infants through high school aged children. As a pediatric audiologist, you will assess hearing and amplification systems through several types of equipment and technologies. You will also work closely with children and parents. Detective-like qualities, strong observation, counseling skills, and a warm personality are an asset to pediatric audiologists.

**Q.** *What do students need to know if they want to pursue an education and/or career in this subject area?*

**A.** Only a handful of audiology and speech–language pathology graduate programs offer significant training in aural habilitation.

# DIVISION 10—ISSUES IN HIGHER EDUCATION

Responses by Richard K. Adler, 2006–2008, Steering Committee Member

**Q.** *How did you become interested in this subject area?*

**A.** I received my Ph.D. because I always wanted to teach at the college/university level. As a new faculty member, I was "green" when it came to understanding the tenure and promotion process, how to balance your personal life with your professional life, how to interact with other academicians, and how to fit in quality research into my hectic teaching schedule. I did not have a mentor to guide me at my first faculty position and I learned by experience. It made sense for me to be an integral part of Division 10 because I wanted to mentor new faculty and do something about the Ph.D. shortage in our discipline.

**Q.** *What does this subject area involve?*

**A.** Division 10 is all about issues in higher education, such as:

1. The Ph.D. shortage—the shortage means there are not enough replacements for those faculty that are retiring and this is a direct threat to the integrity of our academic programs
2. Encouraging master's students to continue studying for the doctorate
3. Infusing evidenced-based practice principles into teaching, clinical practice, and research
4. Infusing multicultural content into academic and clinical experiences
5. Networking with colleagues for new instructional or curriculum ideas
6. Online versus face-to-face versus hybrid delivery of our courses
7. Student engagement in research while balancing our instruction and research projects
8. Mentoring students

9. Collaborative research within speech–language pathology or audiology departments and collaborating with other university departments
10. Mentoring new faculty
11. Faculty keeping up with the latest evidence-based practice while supervising in a university or college clinic

There are many other issues that our members bring up, and Division 10 is there to research the issues and help its members in those areas.

**Q. *What do students need to know if they want to pursue an education and/or career in this subject area?***

**A.** As steering committee members, we would like to encourage students to consider completing a doctoral degree after gaining some clinical experience and then pursuing a career in higher education. Students should realize there is a severe Ph.D. shortage in our discipline. It is a scary prospect sometimes to think about entering academia, but it is a rewarding career and it has its benefits as well as drawbacks like any other job. We encourage students to talk to their professors or anyone in Division 10 and ask questions on how to plan for an academic career or other issues that are pertinent to them. Obtaining a research, teaching, or clinical graduate assistantship will give the student valuable experience of some of the areas involved in an academic career.

# DIVISION 11—ADMINISTRATION AND SUPERVISION

Responses by Shelley J. Victor, 2008–2010, Coordinator

**Q. *How did you become interested in this subject area?***

**A.** I became interested in the area of supervision when I began to supervise speech–language pathology graduate students. My experience is similar to that of the majority of supervisors who do not receive formal academic instruction in supervision. It is assumed that if you are a good clinician, you should therefore be a good supervisor; however, this is not the case. To be effective in the supervisory process, speech–language pathologists need to learn about the process of supervision.

**Q. *What does this subject area involve?***

**A.** Supervision and administration, fields of study although not clinical in nature, need to be grounded in the discipline of communication disorders. A recent publication, *Knowledge and Skills Needed by Speech–Language Pathologists Providing Clinical Supervision* (2008), discusses the skill set that SLPs need to supervise. Supervisors need to be able to develop interpersonal relationships, develop critical thinking skills in their supervisees, develop the supervisee's clinical competence in assessment and intervention, teach the supervisee to self-monitor and self-analyze, and mentor and coach. Administrators may need similar skills depending on the work setting but may also need to be knowledgeable about regulatory and governmental policies and issues; develop budgets and policies; hire, fire, and evaluate personnel. Supervisors and administrators need to be sensitive to individual differences such as race, culture, gender, and age in supervisees.

**Q. *What do students need to know if they want to pursue an education and/or career in this subject area?***

**A.** Although the topic of supervision is discussed in graduate courses, it is unusual that an entire course is devoted to this content. Most professionals who are interested in supervision and administration attend continuing education courses and conferences on the subject, read textbooks and journal articles on the topic, and join Special Interest Division 11. Students who may be interested in this area should consider enrolling in courses that focus on business and human personnel management. Everyone in speech–language pathology is supervised at one point. A supervisee who is armed with knowledge about the supervisory process can ensure that he or she receives an optimal experience.

# DIVISION 12—AUGMENTATIVE AND ALTERNATIVE COMMUNICATION

Responses by Carole Zangari, 2006–2008, Coordinator

**Q. *How did you become interested in this subject area?***

**A.** I have always been interested in extremes and how people cope with challenging situations. Working with people who have the most significant communication challenges has intrigued me since I first met patients with severe aphasia in ninth grade. That interest grew when I was in graduate school at Trenton State College and learned how to make "language boards" in a course on cerebral palsy. (That was pretty progressive for 1982!) It developed into a real passion when I got a chance to apply that information in my clinical externship at a residential facility for children with disabilities. Seeing those kids use language for the first time was an unbelievable experience! In my clinical fellowship (CF), I saw first-hand how using speech-only approaches to communication limited the learning of adults with developmental disabilities. Those approaches not only held them back from developing language but also contributed to frustration. Without a means of expression, people get depressed or angry: that much seemed so clear! Knowing the best ways to teach language and communication to people who were labeled "nonverbal" or "uncommunicative" was a challenge I had not learned much about in graduate school. At an ASHA convention, I met Maryann Romski (now an associate dean for social and behavioral studies at Georgia

State University) and Lyle Lloyd (a professor at Purdue University). Within minutes, I knew that I had to return to graduate school and learn more about this emerging area of augmentative and alternative communication (AAC).

**Q. *What does this subject area involve?***

**A.** AAC involves helping people with the most significant communication difficulties learn to use a variety of tools and strategies to communicate, play, learn language, and develop their literacy skills. It involves working with exciting new technologies. Clinicians with interests in AAC work in a variety of settings, including early intervention, preschools, schools, clinics, hospitals, home health, and skilled nursing facilities. Depending on their specific interests, AAC clinicians may work with individuals who have developmental conditions, such as genetic syndromes or birth injuries, or acquired disorders, such as aphasia, dysarthria, or aphonia.

**Q. *What do students need to know if they want to pursue an education and/or career in this subject area?***

**A.** There are four main things that you have to master to do well as an AAC clinician. First, you have to commit to becoming a skilled clinician who understands how to develop meaningful goals, create effective treatment plans, and implement a range of clinical strategies. It takes years to develop these skills, so you need to be patient with yourself! Next, you have to be comfortable with diversity. AAC covers a wide range of clinical populations, from autism to ALS. While you may choose to specialize in one or two particular disorder areas, most AAC clinicians work with a fairly heterogeneous group of people. You also have to work well in a team. AAC is a field that involves a lot of different disciplines: speech–language pathology, special education, occupational therapy, physical therapy, physiatrist, and others. Finally, you have to embrace a field that changes fairly rapidly. As a relatively new area of intervention, our knowledge of AAC is expanding at an exciting pace.

   To pursue a career in AAC, students should actively steer themselves toward opportunities that will allow them to interact with people who have significant communication challenges. Ask your professors and clinical supervisors for suggestions on where you can observe people with AAC needs. Find out where you can learn more about assistive technology in your community. Share your interest in this population with the instructors who develop clinical schedules and make arrangements for externship placements. There are many wonderful job opportunities for clinical fellowships and experienced clinicians with interests in AAC. Once employed, find out who is most knowledgeable about AAC and seek out skilled and well-respected mentors. Connect with other professionals who have similar interests, through ASHA's Special Interest Divisions, and related professional associations such as International Society for Alternative & Augmentative Communication (ISAAC). Attend

conferences and workshops, both for the information that can be gained
and for the opportunity to network with colleagues.

# DIVISION 13—SWALLOWING AND SWALLOWING DISORDERS (DYSPHAGIA)

Responses by Catriona M. Steele, 2008–2010, Coordinator

**Q. *How did you become interested in this subject area?***

**A.** When I entered graduate school, my primary interest was in aphasia, and
it was a surprise to me to learn that speech–language pathologists also
worked in the area of swallowing. I did not think that I would be very
interested in this area, but my final clinical placement as a student had
a heavy concentration in swallowing, and I quickly learned that I loved
this topic. I particularly love the challenge of trying to understand why
something particular has gone wrong with a patient's swallowing and
then trying to figure out what can be done to help restore functional
swallowing for that patient.

**Q. *What does this subject area involve?***

**A.** This subject area involves learning about the physiology of the swallowing mechanism and its interrelationships with other functions such as
breathing and voice. A huge number of patients experience swallowing
difficulties, and these difficulties can affect patients of all ages, right from
babies in the neonatal intensive care unit (NICU) to very elderly individuals. When patients experience swallowing problems, there are two huge
concerns. The first is safety—can they transport food and liquid through
the mouth and pharynx to the esophagus without aspiration (entry of
material into the airway). The second is efficiency—can they transport
food and liquid to the esophagus in a timely manner so that they meet
their nutritional and hydrational requirements. There are many interventions, either compensatory or rehabilitative, that can be applied to help a
person swallow more safely and efficiently. Understanding the nature of
a person's dysphagia and then matching that to beneficial interventions is
both challenging and rewarding.

**Q. *What do students need to know if they want to pursue
an education and/or career in this subject area?***

**A.** This is probably one of the most medical aspects of our practice. You
should develop competency and comfort both in noninstrumental (clinical) methods of assessment and in instrumental methods such as videofluoroscopy and endoscopy. SLPs are key players on the dysphagia team
but work collaboratively with many other disciplines including medical
specialists (neurologists, radiologists, otolaryngologists, gastroenterolo-
gists, pediatricians, among others), dietitians, and occupational therapists.

There is a huge amount of research ongoing in the field and we are learning more every day. This is an exciting subject area within speech–language pathology that has many opportunities to learn and advance our practice.

## DIVISION 14—COMMUNICATION DISORDERS AND SCIENCES IN CULTURALLY AND LINGUISTICALLY DIVERSE (CLD) POPULATIONS

Responses by Deborah Rhein, 2009–2010, Associate Coordinator

**Q. *How did you become interested in this subject area?***

**A.** I grew up in Central and South America, so I grew up being different than the larger population around me. I also grew up speaking Spanish as a second language, but one that I acquired rather than formally studied. So I guess you could say that thinking about cultural differences and language is something that has always been a part of my life. Later on, I had the opportunity to live in Germany and travel in Europe, which made me even more aware of differing cultural views and how language often reflects those differences.

Once I became an SLP, I spent the majority of my career working with clients whose first language was not English, both children and adults. This led me to a systematic study of the relationships between language, language differences, language disorders, and access to speech–language services. Along the way, I became aware of the need for and passionate about being an advocate for clients from varied cultural and linguistic backgrounds who also have communication disorders.

**Q. *What does this subject area involve?***

**A.** Division 14 exists to promote increased cultural competence and research in a wide range of areas, from advocating awareness of dialectical differences to understanding different views of disability. Appropriate identification and treatment of children with speech and language disorders from different cultural and linguistic backgrounds is a topic frequently sponsored by the division, but the division's mandate is much broader than the second language or second dialect issues. In the recent past, the division has sponsored topics from access to health care for the elderly with different cultural backgrounds to the study of the transgendered voice.

**Q. *What do students need to know if they want to pursue an education and/or career in this subject area?***

**A.** Students need little more than an open mind and a desire to be an advocate for those who may not always have a voice. Through participation in division-sponsored continuing education, they should develop a broad approach to cultural and linguistic diversity. Participation in division-sponsored events and reading of the division newsletter is a great way to develop expertise with clients from culturally and linguistically diverse backgrounds.

# DIVISION 15—GERONTOLOGY

Responses by Paula Zappala, 2008–2010, Steering Committee Member

**Q.** *How did you become interested in this subject?*

**A.** I was first intrigued about the focus of gerontology when I was fortunate enough to perform a 12-week clinical practicum in a skilled nursing facility under the clinical instruction of an SLP who exuded such passion and sincerity with every patient she encountered. With this experience, I found a new interest in the adult population, as prior to this placement I had planned to work in a school setting. In particular, I discovered the wisdom of the older individuals, gaining a new level of respect for the older generations and I had a new appreciation for life. I realized how important it was for our profession to develop our skills and make a positive difference in the lives of all ages alike.

**Q.** *What does this subject area involve?*

**A.** Division 15 focuses on the geriatric population as a whole. This division seeks to provide its subscribers with information and continuing education units (CEUs) opportunities specifically targeting older individuals. While providing professional development opportunities, the main focus is to increase the understanding of the normal and pathological aging process and its effects on communication, cognition, hearing, and swallowing.

**Q.** *What do students need to know if they want to pursue an education and/or career in this subject area?*

**A.** Students should seek the opportunity to observe or have a clinical experience in various settings that provide care to the geriatric population (i.e., home health, active day centers, outpatient, and long-term care). I also recommend that, in each of the care settings, you attempt to visit different companies or facilities to get a good feel for the true care of the geriatric patient. Next, seek these placements by letting your clinical coordinators know your passion is the geriatric population. Many students enter graduate school thinking they want to work with children but realize during clinical that their true interest is geriatrics. Working with this population can be truly rewarding and you can touch many lives.

Students need to know that working with older individuals offers exposure to a wide range and degrees of dysfunctions in various settings. This population offers the SLP autonomy in creating specialized treatment programs and the ability to spend focused quality time with individuals based on the needs of the patient. Speech–language pathologists are able to tailor their career based on their specific interests with this population. The SLP also should realize that working with the older population would frequently involve working with the older individuals' family members and caregivers. It is also a great population to work with if you are interested in being a medical-based SLP who collaborates with other professionals including physicians, nurses, physical therapists, occupational therapists, and nutritionists.

# DIVISION 16—SCHOOL-BASED ISSUES

Responses by Frances K. Block, 2006–2009, Coordinator

**Q.** *How did you become interested in this subject area?*

**A.** Love kids

Love all aspects of speech and language disorders

Love the opportunity to be part of educational and health-related issues

Love a challenge—kids with every kind of disability, syndrome, and health issue are in schools and in speech–language pathology caseloads

Love a dynamic environment—you definitely do not do the same thing every day

Love collaborating

Love advocating for kids

Love the opportunity to learn something new every day

Love the hours, and the school vacations

Love being part of the largest segment of ASHA members—over 50% of ASHA members have chosen to work in schools

**Q.** *What does this subject area involve?*

**A.** Students who want to enter the field of school-based services really must know how to be a "jack or jill of all trades." School-based SLPs must know how to work with children with a wide variety of disabilities and disorders, including children with disorders of fluency, voice, articulation, receptive and expressive language; autism; swallowing disorders; closed-head injury/traumatic brain injury (TBI); children with cochlear implants; reading disabilities, apraxia, augmentative and assistive communication (AAC), congenital syndromes such as Down syndrome, cleft palate, and Fragile X syndrome. Given this broad base of disorders, school-based SLPs must be skilled in a variety of therapy intervention activities and therapy approaches. They must also know how to be team players. This means fitting into the school culture and accepting roles and responsibilities that are not related to direct service delivery. The schools are an exciting and energizing place to work and comprise a work setting that will challenge and stimulate the SLP every day.

**Q. *What do students need to know if they want to pursue an education and/or career in this subject area?***

**A.** In addition to meeting the requirements of the ASHA guidelines, it would be most helpful to do the following:

- Investigate the school certification or licensure requirements within the state(s) where you may want to work, by contacting your state department of education. There are links to every state department of education on the ASHA web site. States may have additional requirements above and beyond what ASHA requires. This may involve extra coursework, and/or tests that must be passed prior to eligibility for a teaching certificate.

- Be aware of timelines for state teacher certification or licensure. Many tests are offered on a limited schedule, with a long period of time before results may be available. Find out everything you need well in advance of your graduation, and plan on how you will be able to schedule meeting all those requirements.

- Schools require collaboration with teachers, support staff, parents, administrators, and others who meet the needs of children. Work on your "people skills" so that you can be an effective team member on an ongoing basis.

- Investigate the various school districts to which you are applying. Most school districts have Web sites with information about salary, benefits, and the community in general. You will be a better interviewee learning some of this information in advance.

- Your education is not finished upon your graduation. Schools not only require SLPs who will continue to learn and grow, but they generally provide many outstanding continuing education opportunities. Continuing education is also required to maintain your ASHA Certificate of Clinical Competence (CCC) and to maintain your professional license and teaching certificate in most states.

- The role of school SLPs has changed greatly over the years. Our role has grown to include how the school-based SLP helps support students and teachers in speech–language and literacy efforts, which includes reading, writing, speaking, and listening.

- If anyone tells you that schools are boring, and that you'll only work with kids with articulation disorders, tell them to join ASHA Division 16, to learn the real truth about how schools are the most exciting places for SLPs to be, and why!

# CONCLUSION

The Divisions provide benefits for both professionals and students. Students are encouraged to take advantage of joining a Division at a discounted rate. Having access to the latest information in your specific special interest will reflect positively on you as a student through your coursework, clinical experiences, thesis or nonthesis project, and so on.

# CHAPTER 27

# Professional Associations in Communication Sciences and Disorders

## INTRODUCTION

Just as the discipline of communication sciences and disorders (CSD) is diverse, so are the associations that support the development, networking, and socialization of CSD professionals. Affiliating with an association is a great way to network with other students and professionals. Joining as a student can be a hefty financial investment, but the rewards of membership are priceless.

## ACADEMY OF APHASIA

Dedicated to research and clinical service, the Academy of Aphasia is a professional organization primarily concerned with language disorders that result from damage to the brain. Associate membership is available for graduate students, postdoctoral fellows, and junior investigators who are interested in the study of language in regard to neurological diseases. The academy holds annual meetings in locations around the globe. More information is available on their Web site (http://academy.angularis.org).

## ACADEMY OF DOCTORS OF AUDIOLOGY

The Academy of Doctors of Audiology (ADA) provides quality resources to private practitioners as well as those who are concerned and interested in quality patient care and business operations. ADA hosts annual conventions, forums, and a student-mentoring program. Students are welcome to join. More information is available on their Web site (http://www.audiologist.org).

## ACADEMY OF NEUROLOGIC COMMUNICATION DISORDERS AND SCIENCES

The Academy of Neurologic Communication Disorders and Sciences (ANCDS) is an organization comprised of speech–language pathologists who strive to promote the enhancement of life and clinical service for individuals with neurological communication disorders. Associated membership for students is available for those interested in networking with professionals who specialize in this area. More information is available on their Web site (http://www.ancds.org).

## ACADEMY OF REHABILITATIVE AUDIOLOGY

The Academy of Rehabilitative Audiology (ARA) works to promote excellence in hearing care with regard to hearing habilitation and rehabilitation services. Student membership is available as well as a research-based scholarships. More information is available on their Web site (http://www.audrehab.org).

## ACOUSTICAL SOCIETY OF AMERICA

The Acoustical Society of America (ASA) is an international society comprised of professionals from multiple disciplines who are interested in the science of sound. Hearing and speech scientists, who are interested in the mechanics of acoustics, are able to participate in this diverse organization. Any graduate or undergraduate student interested in acoustics is allowed to join. Several fellowships, scholarships, grants, and student awards are available for students. More information is available on their Web site (http://asa.aip.org).

## AMERICAN ACADEMY OF AUDIOLOGY

Known as the largest association for audiologists in the world, the American Academy of Audiology (AAA) is devoted to increasing the amount of quality hearing health care. More information is available on their Web site (http://www.audiology.org).

## AMERICAN AUDITORY SOCIETY

The American Auditory Society (AAS) works to expand the understanding and knowledge of ear, hearing, and balance disorders. The society serves as an information pool for hearing and balance disorders, habilitation, rehabilitation, among others. The membership of this organization includes many disciplines and gives professionals a formal way to exchange thoughts, ideas, research, and other findings. Students are welcome to join. Graduate audiology students may complete the graduate student application and receive a complimentary journal subscription. More information is available on their Web site (http://www.amauditorysoc.org).

## AMERICAN CLEFT PALATE–CRANIOFACIAL ASSOCIATION

Comprised of medical professionals from all over the world, the American Cleft Palate–Craniofacial Association (ACPCA) is dedicated to the treatment and study of cleft palates, cleft lips, and other craniofacial defects. The organization strives to create opportunities for communication between the varying disciplines that specialize in this area. Students interested in pursuing future careers that deal with the research and/or service of individuals born with defects of the head and face are encouraged to join. More information is available on their Web site (http://www.acpa-cpf.org).

## AMERICAN SPEECH–LANGUAGE–HEARING ASSOCIATION

Comprised of more than 130,000 members, the American Speech–Language–Hearing Association (ASHA), since its founding in 1925, remains one of the largest and most recognized organizations dedicated to the promotion of speech–language pathology and audiology. ASHA is primarily a professional-only association, which means that students are unable to join. More information about ASHA is available in this guide as well as on the ASHA Web site (http://www.asha.org).

## AMERICAN SPEECH–LANGUAGE–HEARING FOUNDATION

The American Speech–Language–Hearing Foundation (ASHFoundation) supports the research and advancement of the CSD discipline. The organization works to create better lives for those with speech, language, or hearing disorders. The ASHFoundation raises funds annually to support research grants, scholarships for graduate students, clinical recognition awards, among others. There is no student membership for this foundation, but students can apply for their scholarships and other funding opportunities. More information is available on their Web site (http://www.ashfoundation.org).

## ASSOCIATION FOR RESEARCH IN OTOLARYNGOLOGY

The Association for Research in Otolaryngology (ARO) is an international association that is dedicated to research related to ears, head, neck, nose, and anything involving hearing, balance, taste, smell, and so on. Many areas of research are represented, including biochemical, physiological, behavioral, developmental, and evolutionary. Individuals enrolled in a postbaccalaureate degree program related to otolaryngology may join as associate members. More information is available on their Web site (http://www.aro.org).

## COUNCIL OF ACADEMIC PROGRAMS IN COMMUNICATION SCIENCES AND DISORDERS

The Council of Academic Programs in Communicative Sciences and Disorders (CAPCSD) works to assist undergraduate and graduate programs that educate students in CSD. The organization provides information regarding accreditation, curriculum requirements, and funding. More information is available on their Web site (http://www.capcsd.org).

## COUNCIL FOR ACCREDITATION IN OCCUPATIONAL HEARING CONSERVATION

Dedicated to conservation of hearing by enhancing the quality of occupational hearing conservation programs, the Council for Accreditation in Occupational Hearing Conservation (CAOHC) is comprised of members from multiple international associations such as the AAA and the ASHA who are interested in supporting work-related hearing conservation. The CAOHC selects two members from each component organization to serve on the executive council. More information is available on their Web site (http://www.caohc.org).

## EDUCATIONAL AUDIOLOGY ASSOCIATION

The Educational Audiology Association (EAA) is an international professional organization for audiologists that provides a wide range of services for children. These services mainly take place in the educational arena. Student membership is available for audiology students with a bachelor's degree. More information is available on their Web site (http://www.edaud.org).

## INTERNATIONAL SOCIETY OF AUDIOLOGY

The International Society of Audiology (ISA) works toward the advancement of those who are interested in or work in the field of audiology. The society strives to spread information on the prevention and rehabilitation of hearing loss. Student membership is available. More information is available on their Web site (http://www.isa-audiology.org).

## LINGUISTIC SOCIETY OF AMERICA

Primarily comprised of linguistics, the Linguistic Society of America (LSA) is a professional organization interested in promoting the study of language. Any student in the process of completing a degree is eligible for membership. Grants, fellowships, and other valuable resources are available for student members of the society. More information is available on their Web site (http://www.lsadc.org).

## MULTICULTURAL CONSTITUENCY GROUPS

ASHA's Multicultural Constituency Groups were created in order to better serve and provide information for those belonging to or interested in underrepresented minority populations. These groups include the Native American Caucus, the

National Black Association for Speech–Language and Hearing (NBASLH), the Hispanic Caucus, the Asian Indian Caucus, Asian Pacific Islander Caucus, and the Lesbian/Gay/Bisexual Audiologists and Speech–Language Pathologists Caucus. More information can be found on the ASHA Web site. Search for "Multicultural Consistency Groups."

# NATIONAL ACADEMY OF PREPROFESSIONAL PROGRAMS IN COMMUNICATION SCIENCES AND DISORDERS

The National Academy of Preprofessional Programs in Communication Sciences and Disorders (NAPP) is the only organization that is focused on representing undergraduate programs related to communication sciences and disorders. NAPP provides programs with ways to advocate their needs, exchange information, and coordinate self-improvement. Membership into this academy is only for schools. More information is available on their Web site (http://www.calvin.edu/~jvwoude/).

# NATIONAL BLACK ASSOCIATION FOR SPEECH–LANGUAGE AND HEARING

The National Black Association for Speech–Language and Hearing (NBASLH) is an organized group of individuals that strives to network and support the African American community of speech–language pathologists and audiologists. NBASLH accepts members from all ethnic and racial groups. More information is available on their Web site (http://www.nbaslh.org).

# NATIONAL STUDENT SPEECH LANGUAGE HEARING ASSOCIATION

The National Student Speech Language Hearing Association (NSSLHA) is a preprofessional membership association for students interested in the study of CSD. NSSLHA averages 12,000 members and has over 300 local chapters at colleges and universities throughout the United States, Canada, Greece, and Saudi Arabia. NSSLHA is a student-run association, independent of the professional association ASHA. More information can be found in Chapter 24 and on the NSSLHA Web site (http://www.nsslha.org).

# SERTOMA

Sertoma is a nonprofit organization dedicated to "**SER**vice **TO MA**nkind." The organization's primary service projects involve assisting those with speech, hearing, and language disorders. Sertoma has a scholarship program for students. More information is available on their Web site (http://www.sertoma.org).

## SPECIAL INTEREST DIVISIONS

ASHA's Special Interest Divisions (generally referred to as the *Divisions*) comprises 16 specialty areas. Divisions are an affiliate group of ASHA, meaning they have governance and an operating budget separate from ASHA. The Divisions exist for creating a community solely focused on a specialty area. The Divisions are an excellent way for students to connect with professionals who share a similar interest. With national membership in NSSLHA, a student is able to join a Division for $10. More information can be found in Chapter 26 and on the ASHA Web site (search for "Divisions").

## STATE SPEECH AND HEARING ASSOCIATIONS

Many states have their own Speech and Hearing Associations. Each state's association holds information on state regulatory licensing and other important aspects of practicing in that area. Many of these associations welcome student members and hold annual conferences. More information related to your specific state (and others you may be interested in) can be found on the ASHA Web site. Search for "state associations."

## STUDENT ACADEMY OF AUDIOLOGY

The Student Academy of Audiology (SAA) is the national student organization of the AAA. The SAA gives a voice to students pursuing a career in audiology and its related disciplines. There are local SAA chapters on many college and university campuses across the country. More information is available on their Web site (http://www.StudentAcademyofAudiology.org).

## CONCLUSION

Being involved in professional CSD associations is an excellent way for students to develop as preprofessionals. Many of these associations provide students with opportunities to network with other CSD students and professionals, develop leadership skills as future CSD professionals, and provide scholarships/funding for educational cost/research projects. It is highly recommended that students become active members of the associations that apply to them. By being active members, students will be kept well informed about the current issues affecting the CSD discipline.

# APPENDIX A

# Organizational Tools

You will need to be highly organized to succeed as an undergraduate, graduate student, clinician, researcher, and/or professor. Each year you are in school, your organizational needs are likely to increase. Here are some suggestions to help you learn how to be highly organized.

## PURCHASE ORGANIZATIONAL SCHOOL SUPPLIES

- A 1.5- to 2-inch binder for each class (although at the beginning of the semester you can combine several classes into one binder)
- Sticky labels for binders (or a permanent marker to write on binders)
- Dividers and/or Post-it® notes for each class:
  - For regular courses, divide into *syllabus, notes, assignments, handouts,* and *study guides*
  - For clinical courses, divide into *syllabus, notes from lectures, notes from meetings with clinical instructor, to-do-lists to prepare for client sessions, feedback from clinical instructor,* and *handouts*
- Loose-leaf paper for binders
- Spiral or bound notebooks or paper for binders to take notes in each class
- Pen/pencil case to carry supplies to classes
- Pens and pencils
- Highlighters
- Whiteout
- Small Post-It® notes
- Tab dispenser
- Paper clips
- Hole puncher (electric or manual)
- Regular stapler with extra staples
- Labels with your name and e-mail address for all of your textbooks, binders, and planner (you never know when you might lose them)
- Business card paper to create your own business cards

- Personal laminator
- Laminating sheets
- Scissors
- A planner and/or calendar
- Thank-you cards

## PURCHASE USEFUL ELECTRONIC DEVICES AND TOOLS

- Blank CDs (if you have access to a CD writer)
- USB flash drive (remember to back up your files often)
- Personal computer (desktop or laptop) with a word processing program, such as Microsoft® Word
- Printer (if you can afford it, purchase one with a fax, copier, and scanner; there are some affordable models available if you look for them)
- Extra print cartridges
- Extra computer papers
- Internet access (some universities have free Internet access for students)
- Otoscope
- Digital recorder (e.g., for language samples)
- Digital camera (e.g., for making all of those therapy supplies)
- Software to use your digital camera with your computer
- Calculator
- Stop watch or timer (e.g., for timing tests and rates of speech)

## PURCHASE USEFUL FURNITURE

- Desk
- Comfortable desk chair
- Printer cart (if your desk does not have space for a printer)
- Bookcases (for all of your binders and textbooks)
- Bright desk lamp

# APPENDIX B

# Suggested Readings

Bellis, T. J. (2002). *When the brain can't hear: Unraveling the mystery of auditory processing disorder.* New York: Pocket Books.

Brown, C. (1954). *My left foot.* London: Secker & Warburg.

Gannon, J. R. (1981). *Deaf heritage: A narrative history of deaf America.* Silver Spring, MD: National Association of the Deaf.

Keller, H. (1990). *The story of my life.* New York: Bantam.

Keyes, D. (1966). *Flowers for Algernon.* London: Cassell.

Lane, H., Hoffmeister, R., Bahan, B., & Bahan, B. (1996). *A journey into the deaf world.* San Diego, CA: Dawnsign Press.

Murray, F. P., & Goodwillie, S. (1980). *A stutterer's story.* Danville, IL: Interstate Printers & Publishers.

Romoff, A. (2000). *Hear again: Back to life with a cochlear implant.* New York: League for the Hard of Hearing.

Schultz, J. T. (2000). *My walkabout.* Oceanside, CA: Academic Communication Associates.

Sienkiewicz-Mercer, R. (1989). *I raise my eyes to say yes.* Boston: Houghton Mifflin.

Sparks, N. (2000). *The rescue.* New York: Warner Books.

St. Louis, K. O. (2001). *Living with stuttering: Stories, basics, resources, and hope.* Morgantown, WV: Populore.

Thompson, C. E. (1999). *Raising a handicapped child: A helpful guide for parents of the physically disabled.* Oxford, UK: Oxford University Press.

Van Cleve, J., & Crouch, B. (1989). *A place of their own: Creating the Deaf community in America.* Washington, DC: Gallaudet University Press.

# Key Acronyms and Phrases Used in Communication Sciences and Disorders

| | | | |
|---|---|---|---|
| AAA | American Academy of Audiology | CAOHC | Council for Accreditation in Occupational Hearing Conservation |
| AAS | American Auditory Society | | |
| ABD | All but dissertation | CAPCSD | Council of Academic Programs in Communication Sciences and Disorders |
| ACPCA | American Cleft Palate–Craniofacial Association | | |
| ADA | Americans with Disabilities Act | CCC | Certificate of Clinical Competence |
| AIC | Asian Indian Caucus | CEU | Continuing education unit |
| ANCDS | Academy of Neurologic Communication Disorders and Sciences | CF | Clinical fellowship |
| | | CFP | Call for Papers |
| | | CLD | Culturally and linguistically different |
| APA | American Psychological Association | | |
| API | Asian Pacific Islander | CSD | Communication sciences and disorders |
| ARO | Association for Research in Otolaryngology | CV | Curriculum vitae |
| | | DIVISIONS | Special Interest Divisions |
| ASA | Acoustical Society of America | EB | Executive board |
| | | EC | Executive council |
| ASHA | American Speech–Language–Hearing Association | FAFSA | Free Application for Federal Student Aid |
| | | GPA | Grade point average |
| ASHFoundation | American Speech–Language–Hearing Foundation | GSF | Graduate School Fair |
| | | GUR | General university requirement |
| ASL | American Sign Language | IDEA | Individuals with Disabilities Education Act |
| Au.D. | Doctorate of audiology | | |
| BA | Bachelor of arts | IEP | Individual Education Plan |
| BHS | Bachelor of health sciences | IRB | Institutional Review Board |
| | | LC | Legislative council |
| BHSM | Better Hearing and Speech Month | LSA | Linguistic Society of America |
| BS | Bachelor of science | MA | Master of arts |

| | | | |
|---|---|---|---|
| MS | Master of science | OT | Occupational therapist or occupational therapy |
| NAFDA | National Association of Future Doctors of Audiology | PAC | Political Action Committee |
| NAPP | National Academy of Preprofessional Programs in Communication Sciences and Disorders | PET | Positron emission topography |
| | | Ph.D. | Doctorate of philosophy |
| NBASLH | National Black Association for Speech–Language and Hearing | PT | Physical therapist or physical therapy |
| | | Quals | Qualifying examinations |
| | | RC | Regional councilor |
| NBGSA | National Black Graduate Student Association, Inc. | SHS | Speech, language, and hearing scientist |
| NESPA | National Examination in Speech–Language Pathology and Audiology | SLP | Speech–language pathologist |
| NIH | National Institutes of Health | SLP-A/SLPA | Speech–language pathology assistant |
| NSF | National Science Foundation | | |
| NSSLHA | National Student Speech Language Hearing Association | | |

# Index